# Guide to

# Assessment Scales in Bipolar Disorder

## Second Edition

# Guide to

# Assessment Scales in

# Bipolar Disorder

Second Edition

### Eduard Vieta

Director of the Bipolar Disorders Program
Hospital Clinic
University of Barcelona
Spain

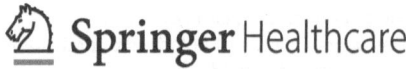 Springer Healthcare

Published by Springer Healthcare Ltd, 236 Gray's Inn Road, London WC1X 8HL, UK

www.springerhealthcare.com

© 2009 Springer Healthcare Ltd, a part of Springer Science+Business Media

First edition 2006
Second edition 2010

British Library Cataloguing in Publication Data.

A catalogue record for this book is available from the British Library.

ISBN 978 1 85873 442 2

Project editor: Lisa Langley
Designers: Taymoor Fouladi and Joe Harvey
Production: Marina Maher

# Contents

**Author biography**     **vii**

1. **Introduction**     **1**

2. **Global assessment scales**     **3**
   Briefly mentioned scales     4
       Global Assessment of Functioning     4
       Clinical Global Impressions for Bipolar Disorder     5
   Featured scale: Clinical Global Impressions for Bipolar Disorder,
   Modified Version     6

3. **Detection of bipolar I**     **9**
   Prevalence of bipolar disorder     9
   Underdiagnosis and misdiagnosis     9
   Implications of misdiagnosis     10
   Improving diagnostic accuracy     11
   Featured scale: Mood Disorder Questionnaire     11

4. **Detection of bipolar II**     **17**
   Featured scale: Bipolar Spectrum Diagnostic Scale     17

5. **Assessment of depression in bipolar disorder**     **23**
   Briefly mentioned scales     23
       Beck Depression Inventory     23
       Montgomery & Asberg Depression Rating Scale     24

6. **Assessment of mania in bipolar disorder**     **27**
   Briefly mentioned scale: Clinician-Administered Rating Scale for Mania     27
   Featured scale: Young Mania Rating Scale     28

7. **Assessment of hypomania**     **33**
   Featured scale: Hypomania Checklist     33

8. **Health-related quality of life assessment in bipolar disorder**     **41**
   Briefly mentioned scales     41
       Medical Outcomes Study Core Survey Instrument     41
       Medical Outcomes Study 20-Item Short-Form Health Survey     42
       Quality of Life Index     42
       32-Item Behavioural and Symptom Identification Scale     43
   Featured scale: EQ-5D/EuroQol     43

9.   **Assessment of pediatric bipolar disorder**                    **47**
     Briefly mentioned scales                                         47
        Child Behaviour Checklist                                     47
        Young Mania Rating Scale-Parent Version                       50
        Children's Global Assessment Scale                            50
     Featured scale: Washington University in St Louis Kiddie Schedule
     for Affective Disorders and Schizophrenia                        50

10.  **Assessment of comorbidities**                                 **69**
     Featured scale: Barcelona Bipolar Eating Disorder Scale          70

11.  **Assessment of functioning**                                   **73**
     Featured scale: Functioning Assessment Short Test                73

12.  **Assessment of suicidality**                                   **77**
     Featured scale: Columbia Classification Algorithm
     of Suicide Assessment                                            78

     **References**                                                   **83**

# Author biography

**Eduard Vieta** is Professor of Psychiatry and the Director of the Bipolar Disorders Program of the Hospital Clinic at the University of Barcelona, Spain. His program is dedicated to providing excellent healthcare for people with bipolar disorder, education and research, and has received worldwide recognition. Professor Vieta also serves as Director of Research at the Clinical Institute of Neuroscience at the same institution and has been an invited Professor at Harvard University, Boston, USA.

Professor Vieta's research focuses on the neurobiology and treatment of bipolardisorder. His programme has been at the forefront of research in the area of emerging treatments, both pharmacological and psychological, including atypicalantipsychotics, antiepileptic drugs, novel compounds, and psychoeducation.Since 2001, his research programme has been funded by the Stanley Medical Research Institute, Bethesda, USA, and he currently leads the Bipolar Research Program at the Spanish Research Network on Mental Disorders, funded by the Spanish Ministry of Science and Innovation. He has made significant contributions to many of the published treatment guidelines on bipolar disorder, including the American Psychiatric Association guidelines and the World Federation of Societies of Biological Psychiatry guidelines.

He has authored more than 300 original articles, over 200 book chapters and 25 books on bipolar disorder. He is also a member of the group on Deconstructing Psychosis for the development of DSM-V. He sits on the editorial board of 16 international scientific journals, including Bipolar Disorders, Journal of Clinical Psychiatry, Psychopathology, Psychotherapy and Psychosomatics, and reviews articles for more than 30 others. He has been the recipient of several international awards for excellence in bipolar disorder including the Aristotle Award in 2005 and the Mogens Schou Award in 2007.

# Author biography

# Chapter 1

# Introduction

Over the past decade, the definition of bipolar disorder has been revised extensively. For many years prior to the revisions, patients with bipolar disorder will have been mistakenly diagnosed as having 'unipolar' depression and treated inappropriately, possibly causing iatrogenic mania. In addition, the concept of '*bipolar spectrum disorder*' has been introduced, with a resultant increase in the estimates of lifetime prevalence, which are considered to be above 5%. These changes have substantial implications for the provision of healthcare and underscore the need to accurately detect and quantify bipolar disorder and its related conditions.

The use of rating scales in bipolar disorders can steer the clinician towards appropriate treatment by:
* helping to establish an accurate diagnosis;
* grading the severity of the condition by quantifying the degree of impairment and disability; and
* characterizing the nature of the symptoms and impairment to enable treatment plans to be tailored to the individual's needs.

This book comprehensively reviews the evaluation of patients with bipolar spectrum disorder. The first chapters evaluate a variety of screening instruments with high sensitivity for detecting bipolar spectrum disorder and a selection of diagnostic scales for specifically diagnosing bipolar disorder or bipolar spectrum disorder. Scales for rating the severity of manic/hypomanic and depressive symptoms are covered in subsequent chapters, as are scales used in the evaluation of impairment, disability and quality of life. The challenges in diagnosing children with bipolar spectrum disorder and the assessment of comorbidities are also explored, and the final two chapters examine functioning and suicidality. Each chapter is prefaced with a summary of key considerations and controversies surrounding the particular area of bipolar disorder or bipolar spectrum disorder under discussion. The scales reviewed herein are by no means exhaustive, but represent the most relevant contemporary scales used in evaluating bipolar spectrum disorder. It is hoped that this book will provide the busy clinician with a selection of useful assessment instruments for pragmatically evaluating the patient with a suspected diagnosis of bipolar disorder.

# Chapter 2

# Global assessment scales

Global rating scales are useful for giving an overall picture of a patient's current status, including information from a wide range of sources and consolidating it in a single measure.

Such global scales may have the following advantages over disease-specific rating scales:
- *The use of more specific rating scales may not capture an accurate picture of the patient's overall condition* – for example, a patient with mania may respond well to treatment and his symptoms, as assessed on a disease-specific scale such as the Young Mania Rating Scale (YMRS), may improve substantially. However, if during treatment for his mania he developed severe depression that stopped him going to work, this would not be captured on the YMRS. A global rating scale may therefore provide a more comprehensive picture of a patient's overall clinical condition than scores on an itemized symptom rating scale, and may be more helpful to clinicians in deciding whether to continue or change a patient's treatment [1].
- *Global rating scales can help clinicians assess whether the results seen on a disease-specific scale are clinically meaningful* – for example, in the early 1990s the Food and Drug Administration (FDA) required a global scale to be included in all trials of antidementia drugs to assess the clinical relevance of changes on scales that measured cognitive function. These global scales, such as the Clinician Interview-Based Impression (CIBI) [2], came with a complete set of guidelines, which helped to ensure interrater reliability plus predictive and content validity.

Global rating scales are sensitive to change and can distinguish drug effects from those of placebo [3]. Thus, they are used extensively in phase II and III drug trials. Perhaps the most widely used is the Clinical Global Impression (CGI) scale, which was first introduced by Guy in 1976 [4]. Both the CIBI and the CGI for Bipolar Disorder (CGI-BP) discussed on page 5 were adapted from this scale.

The original CGI consists of three subscales assessing:
- disease severity;
- change; and
- the therapeutic utility of a treatment which is measured by comparing the therapeutic effect of the drug against any side effects experienced by the patient (the so-called *therapeutic index*).

Guidelines for completing the scale are deliberately left vague to allow the rater maximum flexibility in interpreting the overall response to treatment. A major criticism of disease-specific scales is that statistically significant changes on a particular scale may be of doubtful clinical relevance. The rationale for including global rating scales in clinical trials is that they identify whether a particular treatment confers a clinically meaningful benefit (and not just a statistically significant one). When attempting a global rating in patients with bipolar disorder, there are several challenges to overcome. Firstly, the patient's mood state may vary (eg, they may be manic, depressed, mixed or euthymic), so is an overall rating of disparate mood states valid? Secondly, the clinician will want to know the patient's current clinical status, but he/she will also want to know how well controlled the overall disease is. Can this be achieved with a global rating scale? These issues will be discussed below.

## Briefly mentioned scales

### Global Assessment of Functioning
The *Diagnostic and Statistical Manual of Mental Disorders, fourth edition revised* (DSM-IV-R) [5] describes multi-axial assessment of individuals with mental conditions.

Five axes are described:
- I – Clinical Disorders;
- II – Personality Disorders, Mental Retardation;
- III – General Medical Conditions;
- IV – Psychosocial and Environmental Problems; and
- V – Global Assessment of Functioning.

The scale used to assess the last axis is the Global Assessment of Functioning (GAF). This scale originated as the Health–Sickness rating scale [6], which was later revised to the Global Assessment Scale [7], before being modified to become the GAF [8]. The GAF may be particularly useful in monitoring the progress of an individual in global terms using a single measure. The assessment is limited to psychological, social and occupational functioning, and excludes physical disability and impairment due to environmental limitations. The scale is most frequently used to assess the individual's current level of functioning as this helps to evaluate the need for treatment. However, the GAF can also be used to assess prior levels of functioning (eg, the highest level of functioning over the previous year) or previous functioning over a prescribed period of time (eg, the past year, the preceding 5 years, etc). Some clinicians use the scale at the time of a patient's admission and discharge to allow useful comparisons. The GAF is scored on a scale of 0–100 with anchor points for each decade of scores. Thus, the decade 91–100 represents *'Superior functioning in a wide range of activities, life's problems never seem to get out of hand, is sought out by others because of his or her many positive qualities. No symptoms'*, whereas the decade 11–20 represents *'Some danger of hurting self or others OR occasionally fails to maintain minimal personal hygiene OR gross impairment in communication'*. A score of 0 indicates inadequate information.

In the DSM-IV-R multi-axial assessment system, the GAF score is reported on Axis V as the total score followed by the period to which it applies (eg, GAF = 56 [current]; 82 [highest level in past year]). In relation to bipolar disorder, the GAF has significant limitations. If functioning is impaired, the GAF gives no indication of the cause (mania or depression or a mixed mood state). Furthermore, longitudinal assessments over the previous year may be particularly difficult in patients with rapid-cycling bipolar disorder whose level of functioning may fluctuate dramatically over relatively short periods of time. Although the GAF mixes the assessment of symptoms with that of functioning, some studies have used it to address functional issues only, by which it becomes a more pure and sensitive measurement of functional outcome [9,10].

## Clinical Global Impressions for Bipolar Disorder

As mentioned above, the CGI-BP [11] was developed from the CGI scale of Guy [4]. The original scale was criticized by some authors as being too general to provide meaningful information about a patient's clinical status or the response to treatment [12]. However, others countered that the general nature of the scale meant that any change detected could be regarded as clinically significant. Doubts about the validity and reliability of the scale persisted (because of a lack both of standard definitions of illness severity and change, and of clearly identified timescales for evaluating change). This prompted attempts to standardize the way the CGI is rated in relation to specific mental conditions (eg, dementia or pathological gambling). The CGI-BP is one such scale. As discussed, bipolar disorder can be difficult to assess due to its varied and shifting nature (eg, severity and duration of symptoms, or frequency of different phases). Taking these considerations into account, the CGI was adapted to improve the assessment of patients with bipolar illness. The new CGI-BP allowed for individual assessments of mania, depression and overall bipolar illness, and also assessed the efficacy of both acute treatment and prophylaxis. Precise definitions and guidelines for rating bipolar illness were provided in a CGI-BP user's guide, and the authors anticipated that the reliability and clinical utility of the new scale would be much improved [11].

The CGI-BP consists of three subscales:
- disease severity;
- change in disease severity compared with the preceding phase; and
- change in disease severity compared with the worst phase of the illness.

Each subscale consists of seven items: the severity subscale rates the severity of the current phase from 1 = 'normal, not ill' to 7 = 'very severely ill'; the change subscales rate improvement or deterioration from 1 = 'very much improved' to 7 = 'very much worse' with 4 = 'no change'.

## Featured scale

### Clinical Global Impressions for Bipolar Disorder, Modified Version

The CGI-BP tried to solve the problems posed by the original CGI, but it proved somewhat cumbersome due to the overlapping of concepts (severity and change, general symptoms and manic or depressive symptoms) and the number of evaluations required. The CGI-BP was therefore further refined to give a simpler scale that was more practical to use in clinical trials of new drugs [13]. The Clinical Global Impressions for Bipolar Disorder, Modified Version (CGI-BP-M) is also made up of three subscales.

These assess the severity or 'seriousness' over time of:
• the acute symptoms of depression;
• the acute symptoms of mania; and
• the disease in general.

Unlike the CGI and CGI-BP, the CGI-BP-M dispenses with the direct assessment of change because the CGI severity subscale had more robust interrater reliability than the change subscale [14,15]. If required, a change score can be derived indirectly from the severity score on the CGI-BP-M by subtracting the endpoint severity score from the baseline severity score. Several studies have shown this method of deriving the change score to be sensitive to drug effects [16,17].

Similar to the CGI and CGI-BP, the CGI-BP-M uses a seven-point scale to assess disease severity. In cases where there is a mixed state, the principal score for the severity of acute illness is the higher of the two scores recorded on the mania and depression subscales. If the mean of these two scores were used, this would decrease the overall severity of the mixed state.

# Clinical Global Impressions for Bipolar Disorders, Modified Version

Considering your experience with bipolar patients, how serious is this patient's disease?

| Seriousness of disease | | | | | | |
|---|---|---|---|---|---|---|
| | Normal | Minimum | Mild | Moderate | Pronounced | Serious | Very serious |
| Depression | 1 | 2 | 3 | 4 | 5 | 6 | 7 |
| Mania | 1 | 2 | 3 | 4 | 5 | 6 | 7 |
| General | 1 | 2 | 3 | 4 | 5 | 6 | 7 |

# Chapter 3

# Detection of bipolar I

## Prevalence of bipolar disorder

In recent years, estimates of the lifetime prevalence of bipolar disorder have been extensively revised. Historical rates of 1–2% [1] have now increased to 5–7% [2], although there is widespread variation, with European data indicating a prevalence of 0.6–0.8% [3] and some lifetime estimates of bipolar spectrum disorder as high as 24% [4].

There are two major reasons for the apparent increase in the prevalence rate:
• increased recognition; and
• acceptance of a broader definition of bipolar disorder (so-called 'bipolar spectrum disorder').

In a re-analysis of the US National Epidemiologic Catchment Area (ECA) database, respondents were reclassified according to the presence of features of bipolar spectrum disorder (ie, at least two episodes of subthreshold symptoms of hypomania or mania for at least 1 week). Using these broader criteria, the prevalence rate for bipolar disorder was 6.4% [5]. In contrast, the lifetime prevalence for manic episode (reported two decades previously in the original analysis) was 0.8%, and for hypomania, 0.5%. Thus, subthreshold cases are at least five times more prevalent than DSM-based core syndromal diagnoses.

Caseness can be defined as the level of symptomatology (in terms of both frequency and severity) that is likely to be associated with both suffering or distress in most patients, as well as some degree of functional impairment. The authors contend that, although these subsyndromal patients do not meet current DSM criteria for bipolar disorder, they do fulfill criteria for 'caseness' because they experience high levels of functional impairment, suicidality and utilization of healthcare services.

## Underdiagnosis and misdiagnosis

Supporting evidence for the underdiagnosis and misdiagnosis of bipolar disorder comes from the National Depressive and Manic Depressive Association 2000 survey [6]. More than two-thirds (69%) of respondents with bipolar disorder were misdiagnosed, mostly as suffering from a major depressive disorder (60%), but substantial numbers were also diagnosed as having anxiety disorder (26%), schizophrenia (18%) or personality disorder (17%). One-third of respondents reported that the time between first consultation and accurate diagnosis was 10 years or more. Those who were misdiagnosed consulted an average of four physicians before they were diagnosed correctly and received an average of 3.5 incorrect diagnoses.

In a study of over 34,000 Spanish patients undergoing psychiatric care, including 1153 patients who received a diagnosis of bipolar disorder at least once during at least 10 assessments, it was found that just 30% were given a bipolar disorder diagnosis at the first evaluation and 38% at the last assessment [7]. Only 23% of patients received a bipolar disorder during at least 75% of assessments, of whom 70% received a diagnosis at the first assessment [7]. This compared with 18% of the remaining patients who were diagnosed at the first assessment [7]. Factors associated with diagnostic stability were gender, age at least 40 years, number of psychiatric assessments, and treatment at out-patient mental health centers [7]. However, in samples of hospitalized patients with psychosis, bipolar disorder appears to be the most stable diagnosis [8].

There are several explanations for the frequent misdiagnosis of bipolar disorder. Firstly, many bipolar patients (35–60%) present initially with a major depressive episode [9]. Secondly, many patients with hypomania regard these symptoms as normal or desirable and thus under-report them [10]. Approximately 40% of those initially diagnosed with major depressive disorder have their diagnosis converted to bipolar disorder [11].

## Implications of misdiagnosis

The major consequence of misdiagnosis is inappropriate treatment. Management of bipolar depression with antidepressants alone may induce a manic episode in 30–40% of patients [12]. There is also the risk of inducing rapid cycling with its associated greater treatment resistance and poorer outcome, although less is known about this effect [13]. Current clinical practice guidelines recommend prescribing both antidepressants and mood stabilizers in bipolar patients [14]. Delaying the introduction of a mood stabilizer may increase the risk of lithium resistance (as more bipolar episodes are experienced) [15], suicide [16] and substance abuse [17]. The FDA were sufficiently concerned about the inappropriate use of antidepressants in bipolar patients to include a specific warning in a Public Health Advisory issued in 2004 [18], which states:

*'Because antidepressants are believed to have the potential for inducing manic episodes in patients with bipolar disorder, there is a concern about using antidepressants alone in this population. Therefore, patients should be adequately screened to determine if they are at risk for bipolar disorder before initiating antidepressant treatment so that they can be appropriately monitored during treatment.'*

It is estimated that up to 30% of primary care patients presenting with anxiety or depressive symptoms will have a bipolar spectrum disorder [19,20]. Thus, there is an urgent need to improve the diagnosis of these conditions in primary care. Screening tools such as the Mood Disorder Questionnaire (MDQ) may prove particularly beneficial.

## Improving diagnostic accuracy

There are several important factors that can help improve the diagnosis of bipolar disorder. Increased awareness of the pitfalls in diagnosis can help clinicians to avoid them. Patients may not appreciate the pathological significance of hypomanic symptoms, so clinicians should ask specific questions to all patients presenting for the first time with an episode of depression. It is important to ask about a past history of manic/hypomanic symptoms (especially the occurrence of hypomania after depressive episodes) as well as evaluating whether such symptoms are currently present. A collateral history from a close friend or relative should also be sought as it is frequently revealing.

There are several features of bipolar depression that help distinguish it from 'unipolar' depression (ie, major depressive disorder) [21,22] and these should be sought in the history and examination:

- early age at onset of episodes;
- sudden onset of episodes;
- brief duration;
- history of antidepressant-induced mania;
- history of postpartum depression;
- presence of psychosis;
- presence of psychomotor retardation;
- presence of atypical features such as hypersomnia; and
- family history of bipolar disorder or 'loaded' pedigrees (ie, extensive family history of mental health problems).

For the busy physician with limited time, a screening questionnaire such as the MDQ can be very useful. Not only does it provide an overall score that can be used to assess the probability of bipolar disorder, but it also identifies specific symptoms (which the physician can further elaborate) and the degree of functional impairment experienced by the patient during symptomatic episodes. Such screening instruments can also enhance clinician–patient communication by providing a focus for subsequent discussion.

# Featured scale

## Mood Disorder Questionnaire

The MDQ is a screening instrument for bipolar disorder. It does not distinguish between the different types of bipolar disorder, but is probably most sensitive at detecting bipolar I disorder. It may have particular clinical utility in primary care where it can aid the busy clinician in identifying those patients at highest risk of having bipolar disorder. Patients who screen positive on the MDQ should then receive a complete clinical assessment for bipolar spectrum disorder. The MDQ can be completed by the patient or clinical staff in under 5 minutes.

There are three sections:
• a symptom checklist;
• a question asking whether any symptoms experienced occurred during the same period of time; and
• an evaluation of the functional impairment associated with these symptoms.

The symptom checklist consists of 13 questions to be answered by a 'yes' or 'no', which are derived from DSM-IV criteria for mania and hypomania. The MDQ screens for a lifetime history of manic or hypomanic symptoms.

In the original validation study of the MDQ [23] (performed on 198 tertiary care psychiatric outpatients), a screening score of 7 or more out of 13 was chosen as the optimal cut-off, as it provided good sensitivity (0.73) and very good specificity (0.90). Thus, by using this threshold, seven out of ten people with a bipolar spectrum disorder would be correctly identified, and three out of ten would be missed (ie, three false negatives).

Similarly, in those who did not have a bipolar spectrum disorder, nine out of ten would be successfully screened out, and one out of ten would be a false positive. Estimates of sensitivity and specificity in subsequent studies have varied considerably. A postal survey in the general population found a much lower sensitivity (0.28), but a higher specificity (0.97) than the original [24]. Another study in psychiatric outpatients estimated sensitivity and specificity as 0.58 and 0.67, respectively. In this study, sensitivity was higher in bipolar I patients (0.69) compared with either bipolar II disorder or bipolar disorder not otherwise specified (NOS) (0.30) [25]. However, omitting question 3 (ie, not taking functional impairment as a criterion for a positive test) increased sensitivity from 0.58 to 0.78.

The MDQ has also been studied in a UK sample, in which 54 bipolar spectrum disorder patients and 73 unipolar depressive disorder patients were administered the questionnaire [26]. Using the original cutoff guidelines, the overall sensitivity was 0.76, at 0.83 for bipolar I disorder and 0.67 for bipolar II disorder [26]. The specificity was 0.86 and the overall positive and negative predictive values were 0.80 and 0.83, respectively [26]. Re-running the analysis using only Section 1 and an optimal cutoff of nine symptom items, the results indicated improvements in sensitivity for both bipolar I and bipolar II disorder, at 0.90 and 0.88, respectively [26]. There was a slight improvement in specificity, at 0.90, while the overall positive and negative predictive values were 0.79 and 0.92, respectively [26].

A French version of the MDQ was administered to 96 outpatients suffering from mood disorders, of whom 54 had been diagnosed with bipolar disorder on the Structured Clinical Interview for DSM-IV, and again 1 month later [27]. The MDQ had a sensitivity of 74.1% (90.3% for bipolar I disorder and 52.4% for bipolar II disorder) and a specificity of 90.5% at a cut-off score of 7 or more [27]. The questionnaire had adequate internal consistency, at a Cronbach alpha of 0.89, and test–reliability, at a kappa coefficient of 0.79 [27]. Stability was similar for both bipolar I and II disorder [27]. Another analysis of the French version of the MDQ in 44 bipolar spectrum disorder patients and 102 unipolar disorder patients in Switzerland indicated that the MDQ has reasonable test–retest reliability and screening for bipolar disorder is largely independent of depression severity [28].

In order to test a Spanish version of the MDQ, a total of 62 bipolar I disorder patients, 52 bipolar II disorder patients, 58 major depression patients, and 60 healthy controls, who were administered the questionnaire on two occasions 4 weeks apart [29]. For the detection of bipolar disorder, the MDQ, at a cutoff of at least seven positive responses, had a sensitivity of 60% and a specificity of 0.98, and positive and negative probability ratios of 35.5 and 2.4, respectively [29]. Interestingly, if only seven positive responses was used as the cutoff, the sensitivity and specificity rose to 0.81 and 0.95, respectively, while the positive and negative probability quotients were 16 and 5.3 [29]. The Spanish version of the MDQ has been successfully used in a recent diagnostic screening study in patients with depression [30].

A Finnish translation of the MDQ was used to screen 109 consecutive nonschizophrenic psychiatric out- and inpatients in Espoo, Finland, in a pilot study for the Jorvi Bipolar Study (JoBS) [31]. Sensitivity of the questionnaire was increased to 0.90 if minor functional impairment was included as a positive screening factor (the authors argue that this increases the probability of detecting bipolar II patients, who in general are not substantially functionally impaired). However, specificity in this study was low and only 53% of the patients who screened positive on the MDQ were diagnosed as having bipolar disorder on the Structured Clinical Interview for DSM-IV (SCID). Of these, 70% of type I patients had previously been diagnosed correctly, compared with a rate of 20% in type II patients. These results underscore the usefulness of the MDQ as a screening instrument.

A total of 185 psychiatric outpatients primarily being treated for mood disorders were studied to test the validity of a Chinese version of the MDQ. Forty eight patients had bipolar I disorder, nine had bipolar II disorder, five had bipolar disorder not otherwise specified, 35 had depressive disorder, one had substance dependence, and four were unaffected by mood or substance use disorders [32]. Using a criteria of seven or more symptoms causing either moderate or serious problems, the sensitivity of the MDQ was low, at 0.45, and the specificity was 0.93 [32]. The positive and negative predictive values were 0.93 and 0.53, respectively. When the impairment criterion was omitted, the sensitivity and specificity of the questionnaire were improved, at 0.73 and 0.88, respectively, while the positive and negative predictive values were 0.90 and 0.67, respectively [32].

In addition, Turkish and Persian versions of the MDQ have been validated [33, 34]. For the Turkish version, which was tested in 309 psychiatric outpatients, the greatest sensitivity was achieved with a cutoff of five positive responses, at 0.81, while the greatest specificity was seen with a cutoff of seven positive responses, at 0.77 [33]. Administering the Persian version of the MDQ to 188 outpatients, the researchers found that, at a cutoff score of five, the sensitivity was 0.63, the specificity was 0.71, the positive predictive value was 0.78 and the negative predictive value was 0.53 [34].

## Limitations of the MDQ
Many patients with bipolar II disorder consider their hypomanic periods to be normal phases of especially productive activity and thus may fail to recognize them as episodes of abnormally expansive mood. The MDQ may fail to detect this symptom and thus may provide a false-negative screening result. Other scales are perhaps more sensitive for detecting bipolar II disorder.

Many clinicians view the occurrence of treatment-emergent hypomania/mania as being of important diagnostic value when considering bipolar I disorder. However, this event is not considered in either the MDQ or DSM-IV. A family history of bipolar disorder is frequently lacking because of the considerable underdiagnosis of the disorder. Instead, there may be a family history of depression, anxiety, alcohol and/or substance abuse or antisocial behavior.

# The Mood Disorder Questionnaire

Rater:................................................................   Date: ......................................

## Patient's personal details

Name: .................................................................   Age: ............   Gender: M/F

| | Yes | No |
|---|---|---|
| **1.** Has there ever been a period of time when you were not your usual self and... | | |
| ...you felt so good or so hyper that other people thought you were not your normal self or you were so hyper that you got into trouble? | ☐ | ☐ |
| ...you were so irritable that you shouted at people or started fights or arguments? | ☐ | ☐ |
| ...you felt much more self-confident than usual? | ☐ | ☐ |
| ...you got much less sleep than usual and found you didn't really miss it? | ☐ | ☐ |
| ...you were much more talkative or spoke faster than usual? | ☐ | ☐ |
| ...thoughts raced through your head or you couldn't slow your mind down? | ☐ | ☐ |
| ...you were so easily distracted by things around you that you had trouble concentrating or staying on track? | ☐ | ☐ |
| ...you had much more energy than usual? | ☐ | ☐ |
| ...you were much more active or did many more things than usual? | ☐ | ☐ |
| ...you were much more social or outgoing than usual (eg, you telephoned friends in the middle of the night)? | ☐ | ☐ |
| ...you were much more interested in sex than usual? | ☐ | ☐ |
| ...you did things that were unusual for you or that other people might have thought were excessive, foolish or risky? | ☐ | ☐ |
| ...spending money got you or your family into trouble? | ☐ | ☐ |

**2.** If you checked YES to more than one of the above, have several of these ever     Yes    No
happened during the same period of time? *Please circle one response only.*

**3.** How much of a problem did any of these cause you (eg, being unable to work;
having family, money or legal troubles; getting into arguments or fights)?
*Please circle one response only.*

| No problem | Minor problem | Moderate problem | Serious problem |

© Hirschfeld RMA, Williams JB, Spitzer RL *et al.* **Development and validation of a screening instrument for bipolar spectrum disorder: the Mood Disorder Questionnaire.** *Am J Psychiatry* 2000; **157**:1873–1875.

# Detection of bipolar II

Although bipolar II disorder is generally viewed as a mild form of manic–depressive illness, the frequency of episodes, comorbidity rates, functional impairment and suicidality may be even higher than in bipolar I disorder [1].

The definition of bipolar disorder is likely to evolve further, but two important recent revisions to the diagnostic criteria relate to the duration of hypomanic episodes and the inclusion of 'softer' criteria. Currently, according to DSM-IV-R, a diagnosis of hypomania requires symptoms to be present for at least 4 days [2]. There is a strong case being made for reducing this duration even further, to avoid ignoring hypomanic episodes of shorter duration and thus mistakenly diagnosing a patient with 'unipolar' rather than bipolar depression [3]. Such erroneous diagnoses can lead to inappropriate treatment, which puts patients at risk. The second diagnostic revision relates to the concept of 'bipolar spectrum disorders'. This is an evolving concept but essentially is viewed as a longitudinal history of mood swings. These mood swings may also include mixed states (simultaneous mania and depression) and hyperthymic temperament (cheerful, exuberant, meddlesome, uninhibited, overconfident, grandiose) as well as the more easily diagnosed mania, hypomania and major depression [4].

The mean modal duration of hypomania is 1–3 days [5]. Thus, current DSM-IV criteria for bipolar disorder underdiagnose bipolar II disorder [6]. Most bipolar patients have the type II disorder, therefore it is likely that many patients are either undiagnosed or misdiagnosed as having unipolar depression (ie, major depressive disorder). As discussed in the previous chapter, the diagnosis of bipolar II disorder has undergone extensive revision and is continuing to evolve. There is much discussion about how far the spectrum of bipolar disorders extends and where the divide between normality and abnormality resides. If the diagnostic criterion relating to the duration of hypomania is reduced from 4 days to 1 day, many more patients would qualify for a diagnosis of bipolar spectrum disorder. The scale described below is more sensitive to the detection of bipolar II disorder than the MDQ.

## Featured scale

### Bipolar Spectrum Diagnostic Scale
The Bipolar Spectrum Diagnostic Scale (BSDS) is a screening instrument for bipolar spectrum disorder that is more sensitive to bipolar II disorder than the MDQ. It is a narrative account of 19 features that may occur in people with bipolar disorder. The narrative is read by the patient who then rates it for overall applicability to their particular situation, before rating each item of the narrative. A total score is obtained which can then be used

to evaluate the probability that bipolar spectrum disorder is present. This style of evaluation is designed to capture the more subtle features of bipolar II disorder.

The scale was originally created by Dr Ronald Pies [7] and then further revised and field tested by Drs Nassir Ghaemi and Chris Miller [8] who compared it with the MDQ. In this research, the MDQ was administered to 37 patients with bipolar disorder, and the BSDS to 73 patients with bipolar disorder and 20 patients with unipolar illness. The results on all scales were compared with clinicians' DSM-IV-based diagnoses. The overall sensitivity of the BSDS was 0.81 and was similar in both bipolar I and bipolar II patients (0.77 each). Specificity was high (0.85) when the scale was used in unipolar depressed patients. The MDQ was more sensitive for bipolar I than bipolar spectrum illness, whereas the BSDS was highly sensitive and specific for bipolar spectrum illness.

A cut-off score of 13 was identified as the optimal balance of sensitivity and specificity, and this can be used to signify 'caseness'. However, the scale can also be scored in terms of probability, as shown in the table below.

| Interpretation of the Bipolar Spectrum Diagnostic Scale score | |
|---|---|
| Score | Likelihood of bipolar disorder |
| 0–6 | Highly unlikely |
| 7–12 | Low probability |
| 13–19 | Moderate probability |
| 20–25 | High probability |

In another study led by Nassir Ghaemi, 44 patients with bipolar I disorder, three with bipolar II disorder, 21 with bipolar disorder not otherwise specific and 27 patients with unipolar major depressive disorder were administered the BSDS [9]. The overall sensitivity of the BSDS for diagnosing bipolar disorder was 0.76, at 0.75 for bipolar I disorder and 0.79 for bipolar II disorder/bipolar disorder not otherwise specified [9]. The overall specificity was 0.85 [9]. While lowering the cutoff score from 13 to 12 had minimal effect on the sensitivity of the BSDS, reducing it to 0.75 from 0.76, there was a large decrease in specificity, down to 0.85 from 0.93 [9].

A Persian version of the BSDS has been tested in 181 psychiatric outpatients, of whom 103 had bipolar I disorder, 38 had major depressive disorder, 25 had psychotic disorders, 10 had other bipolar disorders, and three had other depressive disorders [10]. Using a cutoff score of 14, the researchers found that the sensitivity and specificity of the BSDS was 0.52 and 0.79, while a cutoff of 13 increased the sensitivity by 0.05 and reduced the specificity by 0.07 [10].

Patients identified with probable or possible bipolar disorder should undergo a comprehensive diagnostic evaluation; for example, using a recognized diagnostic system such as the Structured Clinical Interview for DSM-V (SCID), and obtaining a collateral history from a close friend or family member.

# Bipolar Spectrum Diagnostic Scale

Rater: ................................................................    Date: ....................................

## Patient's personal details

Name: ................................................................    Age: ............    Gender: M/F

> **Instructions:**
> Please read through the entire passage below before filling in any blanks.

1. Some individuals notice that their mood and/or energy levels shift drastically ☐
   from time to time

2. These individuals notice that, at times, their mood and/or energy level is ☐
   very low, and at other times, very high

3. During their 'low' phases, these individuals often feel a lack of energy, ☐
   a need to stay in bed or get extra sleep, and little or no motivation to do
   things they need to do

4. They often put on weight during these periods ☐

5. During their low phases these individuals often feel 'blue', sad all the time ☐
   or depressed

6. Sometimes during these low phases, they feel hopeless or even suicidal ☐

7. Their ability to function at work or socially is impaired ☐

8. Typically, these low phases last for a few weeks, but sometimes they last ☐
   only a few days

9. Individuals with this type of pattern may experience a period of 'normal' ☐
   mood in between mood swings, during which their mood and energy levels
   feel 'right' and their ability to function is not disturbed

10. They may then notice a marked shift or 'switch' in the way they feel ☐

11. Their energy increases above what is normal for them, and they often get ☐
    many things done they would not ordinarily be able to do

12. Sometimes, during these 'high' periods, these individuals feel as if they ☐
    have too much energy or feel 'hyper'

13. Some individuals, during these high periods, may feel irritable, 'on edge' ☐
    or aggressive

14. Some individuals, during these high periods, take on too many activities at once ☐

15. During these high periods, some individuals may spend money in ways that cause them trouble ☐

16. They may be more talkative, outgoing or sexual during these periods ☐

17. Sometimes, their behavior during these high periods seems strange or annoying to others ☐

18. Sometimes, these individuals get into difficulty with coworkers or the police during these high periods ☐

19. Sometimes, they increase their alcohol or nonprescription drug use during these periods ☐

> Now that you have read this passage, please tick one of the following four boxes:
>
> ☐ This story fits me very well, or almost perfectly
>
> ☐ This story fits me fairly well
>
> ☐ This story fits me to some degree, but not in most respects
>
> ☐ This story doesn't really describe me at all

Now please go back and put a tick after each sentence (numbered 1–19 above) that definitely describes you.

---

**Scoring:**

Each sentence ticked is worth one point. Then, to this score add the following (depending upon which of the above four boxes you ticked):

| | |
|---|---|
| • Add 6 points if you ticked 'fits me very well or almost perfectly' | 6 |
| • Add 4 points if you ticked 'fits me fairly well' | 4 |
| • Add 2 points if you ticked 'fits me to some degree, but not in most respects' | 2 |
| • Add 0 points if you ticked 'doesn't really describe me at all' | 0 |

**Your total score** .....

**Likelihood of bipolar disorder:**

0–6     Highly unlikely
7–12    Low probability
13–19   Moderate probability
20–25   High probability

**Optimum threshold for positive diagnosis:** score of 13 or above.

© Pies R. **Bipolar Spectrum Diagnostic Scale validation study.** Paper presented at: *American Psychiatric Association 155th Annual Meeting,* Philadelphia, USA; 2002.

# Chapter 5

# Assessment of depression in bipolar disorder

Up to 60% of bipolar patients initially present with depression [1], and the majority of bipolar patients will experience a major depressive episode at some stage in their lives. Depressive symptoms have the greatest negative impact on the lives of patients with bipolar disease [2,3]. If depression is suspected, the use of rating scales can aid the diagnosis (by ensuring that all key symptoms are addressed), quantify the severity of depression and assist in monitoring the response to treatment. Their use also optimizes a consistent therapeutic approach in successive evaluations.

In the past, the evaluation of depression has received much more attention than that of mania and there is broad clinical experience in the use of depression rating scales. The characteristics of three of the most commonly used scales are discussed below, although much of the experience comes from their use in unipolar depression.

## Briefly mentioned scales

### Beck Depression Inventory
The Beck Depression Inventory (BDI) [4] is one of the oldest and has become the most widely used depression-rating scale since its introduction in 1961. It has been used extensively in clinical trials. It was originally developed to assist the evaluation of depression in psychotherapy patients [5] and not surprisingly, there is therefore an emphasis on cognitive symptoms (33% of its variance is directed to cognitive symptoms, but only 14% to mood and/or anhedonia) [6].

The BDI is a 21-item self-administered scale that takes about 10 minutes to complete. It can be used as a screening tool and has been shown to discriminate effectively between depressed and nondepressed individuals. It is useful for monitoring response to treatment, but is less effective at gauging the severity of a depressive episode [7]. It has been used scantly in bipolar research. The inventory covers a range of somatic, cognitive, affective and behavioral symptoms associated with depression. Each item consists of four statements that describe a particular symptom, increasing in severity with each subsequent statement. The patient is instructed to read each group of statements and identify the single statement that best describes the way they have felt during the past week. Each item is rated on a scale of 0 (absent/normal) to 3 (most severe), giving a maximum score of 63. Scores of 18 or greater are considered to be indicative of significant depression (see table on page 24).

| Suggested scoring system for Beck Depression Inventory | |
|---|---|
| **Score** | **Comment** |
| 1–10 | These ups and downs are considered normal |
| 11–16 | Mild mood disturbance |
| 17–20 | Borderline clinical depression |
| 21–30 | Moderate depression |
| 31–40 | Severe depression |
| >40 | Extreme depression |

To examine the ability of the BDI to measure self-reported depression in bipolar I disorder patients, 120 outpatients, of whom one third had recently experienced manic, mixed, or depressive episodes, were administered the questionnaire [8]. As expected, patients with depressed episodes had significantly higher BDI scores than those with mixed episodes, who in turn had significantly higher scores than patients with manic episodes, at average scores of 34.1, 25.9, and 11.7, respectively [8]. The questionnaire also demonstrated good to excellent internal consistency [8].

## Montgomery and Asberg Depression Rating Scale

The Montgomery and Asberg Depression Rating Scale (MADRS) [9] is a 10-item depression rating scale, administered by a trained interviewer, which takes about 15–20 minutes to complete. It was originally designed to be sensitive to change so that it could be used in studies of treatments for depression. As a result, it has been used widely in clinical trials of antidepressant medication for quantitative evaluation and assessment of changes in symptoms. Its ease of use and good interrater reliability enable nursing staff as well as physicians to use the scale. Specific guidelines on the use of the scale optimize interrater reliability. It has been translated into a variety of languages.

The ten items of the scale are:
- apparent sadness;
- reported sadness;
- inner tension;
- reduced sleep;
- reduced appetite;
- concentration difficulties;
- lassitude;
- inability to feel;
- pessimistic thoughts; and
- suicidal thoughts.

There is a relative lack of emphasis on somatic symptoms compared with other depression rating scales, making it particularly useful for the assessment of depression in people with physical illnesses. Each item is rated on a seven-point scale (scores of 0–6). Anchor points are provided for scores of 0, 2, 4 and 6. The maximum total score is 60. Various cut-off scores have been suggested [10] but the most recent are presented in the table below [11].

| Suggested scoring system for MADRS | |
| --- | --- |
| **Score** | **Comment** |
| 0–8 | No depression/recovered |
| 9–17 | Mild depression |
| 18–34 | Moderate depression |
| ≥35 | Severe depression |

# Chapter 6

# Assessment of mania in bipolar disorder

In previous chapters we have discussed the use of screening to detect patients who may have bipolar disorder. Once such high-risk patients are identified, it is necessary to confirm the diagnosis using recognized international diagnostic criteria (DSM-IV-R [1] or *International Statistical Classification of Diseases and Health-Related Problems*, 10th revision [ICD-10] [2]).

If mania or hypomania is present (or suspected), the use of the mania rating scales described below can assist in both confirming the diagnosis and quantifying the severity of the condition. Another important use of these rating scales is to monitor the patient's response to therapeutic interventions.

The chief advantage of the Young Mania Rating Scale (YMRS) is that it has been used extensively in clinical trials and it is therefore likely to remain the gold standard scale for rating mania for the foreseeable future. However, further study is required to translate changes in ratings into clinically meaningful effects. In addition, the relative weighting attached to individual scale items needs further evaluation [3].

## Briefly mentioned scale

### Clinician-Administered Rating Scale for Mania
The Clinician-Administered Rating Scale for Mania (CARS-M) [4] has several uses:
- to assess the severity of a manic episode, including psychotic symptoms;
- to assist diagnosis by identifying the presence of manic symptoms (individual items correspond to DSM-IV diagnostic criteria for mania); and
- to assess response to antimanic treatment in clinical trials.

The CARS-M is a 15-item scale. The time period for assessing symptoms is usually over the previous 7 days, although this may be shortened for clinical research, if necessary. Most items are scored from 0 (absent) to 5. It contains two subscales, the mania subscale and the psychotic/disorganization subscale, each of which should be scored separately. The mania subscale score is derived by summing the scores for items 1–10. The severity of mania can be gauged using the cut-off limits shown in the table on the next page.

| Suggested scoring system for CARS-M | |
|---|---|
| **Score** | **Comment** |
| 0–7 | None or questionable mania |
| 8–15 | Mild mania |
| 16–25 | Moderate mania |
| ≥26 | Severe mania |

The psychotic/disorganization subscale is derived by summing items 11–15. Combining both subscale scores gives a global measure of 'mania with psychotic features', but only the mania subscale score should be used to provide an overall rating of mania. Use of two subscales permits the separate assessment of manic and psychotic symptoms, which may respond differently to treatment.

The CARS-M takes approximately 15–30 minutes to administer. Raters are encouraged to receive training in the use of the scale prior to using it. The tool has been translated into Spanish and Portuguese.

The CARS-M represents an improvement over previous scales in that the norm was based on a much larger patient sample (n=96) and across all major diagnostic categories (schizophrenia, schizoaffective disorder, bipolar disorder and major depression). It has good internal validity and test–retest reliability (0.93). Additional benefits include the standardized interview format and guidelines describing its use, scoring and administration.

# Featured scale

## Young Mania Rating Scale
The YMRS [4] is a reliable and valid rating scale, and one of the most widely used assessment instruments in clinical trials of antimanic agents.

The major drawbacks of the scale are that:
• it assesses only manic symptoms (there are no items assessing depression);
• it may be difficult to administer in patients who are highly thought disordered; and
• it may not be as sensitive for mild forms of mania, such as hypomania.

The YMRS is an 11-item clinician-administered rating scale used to assess the severity of mania for either clinical or research purposes. The interviewer explores each of the scale items with the patient and the patient is asked to base his/her answers on their experiences during the previous 48 hours. The scale is scored by the interviewer based on the subjective reports of the patient, coupled with the interviewer's own observations of the patient's behavior during the interview. The objective observations are afforded greater weight than the patient self-report. The scale takes about 15–30 minutes to complete. Each item has operationally defined anchor points and is usually scored on a scale of 0–4. However, four of the items (irritability, speech, content and disruptive–aggressive behavior) are given twice the weight of the other seven in an attempt to compensate for poor cooperation from severely ill patients.

The minimum score is 0 and the maximum is 60. In mania trials, scores of 20 or greater are commonly required for inclusion. Following treatment, patients scoring 12 or less are considered to be in remission [5], but 12 has also been used as a threshold for hypomania and the absence of hypomania should not be considered the same as clinical remission. In fact, more restrictive definitions of remission, such as scoring 7 or less, have also been used in several studies [6,7]. Other definitions of response include a decrease from baseline YMRS score of 33% or 50%.

The scale demonstrates good interrater reliability. In the original validation study, there was a high correlation between the scores of two independent clinicians on both the total score (0.93) and the individual item scores (0.66–0.92) [8]. The total score also correlated highly with an independent global rating, with the scores on two other mania rating scales administered at the same time, and with the length of subsequent hospital stay for each patient. In addition, the scale was able to distinguish levels of severity based on global ratings and revealed treatment effects. It is this sensitivity to change that makes the YMRS a suitable scale for use in clinical trials in the treatment of mania.

# Young Mania Rating Scale (Clinician Administered)

Rater: ..................................................................   Date: ....................................

## Patient's personal details

Name: ..............................................................   Age: ............   Gender: M/F

---

**Guide for scoring items:**

The purpose of each item is to rate the severity of that abnormality in the patient. When several keys are given for a particular grade of severity, the presence of only one is required to qualify for that rating.

The keys provided are guides. One can ignore the keys if that is necessary to indicate severity, although this should be the exception rather than the rule.

Scoring between the points given (whole or half points) is possible and encouraged after experience with the scale is acquired. This is particularly useful when severity of a particular item in a patient does not follow the progression indicated by the keys.

---

1. **Elevated mood**

| | |
|---|---|
| Absent | 0 |
| Mildly or possibly increased on questioning | 1 |
| Definite subjective elevation, optimistic, self-confident, cheerful, appropriate to content | 2 |
| Elevated, inappropriate to content, humorous | 3 |
| Euphoric, inappropriate laughter, singing | 4 |

2. **Increased motor activity energy**

| | |
|---|---|
| Absent | 0 |
| Subjectively increased | 1 |
| Animated, gestures increased | 2 |
| Excessive energy, hyperactive at times, restless (can be calmed) | 3 |
| Motor excitement, continuous hyperactivity (cannot be calmed) | 4 |

3. **Sexual interest**

| | |
|---|---|
| Normal, not increased | 0 |
| Mildly or possibly increased | 1 |
| Definite subjective increase on questioning | 2 |
| Spontaneous sexual content, elaborates on sexual matters, hypersexual by self-report | 3 |
| Overt sexual acts (towards patients, staff or interviewer) | 4 |

### 4. Sleep

| | |
|---|---|
| Reports no decrease in sleep | 0 |
| Sleeping less than normal amount by up to 1 hour | 1 |
| Sleeping less than normal by more than 1 hour | 2 |
| Reports decreased need for sleep | 3 |
| Denies need for sleep | 4 |

### 5. Irritability

| | |
|---|---|
| Absent | 0 |
| Subjectively increased | 2 |
| Irritable at times during the interview, recent episodes of anger or annoyance on ward | 4 |
| Frequently irritable during interview, short and curt throughout | 6 |
| Hostile, uncooperative, interview impossible | 8 |

### 6. Speech (rate and amount)

| | |
|---|---|
| No increase | 0 |
| Feels talkative | 2 |
| Increased rate or amount at times, verbose at times | 4 |
| Push, consistently increased rate and amount, difficult to interrupt | 6 |
| Pressured, uninterruptible, continuous speech | 8 |

### 7. Language–thought disorder

| | |
|---|---|
| Absent | 0 |
| Circumstantial, mild distractibility, quiet thoughts | 1 |
| Distractible, loses goal of thoughts, changes topic frequently, racing thoughts | 2 |
| Flight of ideas, tangentiality, difficult to follow, rhyming, echolalia | 3 |
| Incoherent, communication impossible | 4 |

### 8. Content

| | |
|---|---|
| Normal | 0 |
| Questionable plans, new interests | 2 |
| Special project(s), hyperreligious | 4 |
| Grandiose or paranoid ideas, ideas of reference | 6 |
| Delusions, hallucinations | 8 |

### 9. Disruptive–aggressive behavior

| | |
|---|---|
| Absent, cooperative | 0 |
| Sarcastic, loud at times, guarded | 2 |
| Demanding, threats on ward | 4 |
| Threatens interviewer, shouting, interview difficult | 6 |
| Assaultative, destructive, interview impossible | 8 |

### 10. Appearance

| | |
|---|---|
| Appropriate dress and grooming | 0 |
| Minimally unkempt | 1 |
| Poorly groomed, moderately dishevelled, overdressed | 2 |
| Dishevelled, partly clothed, garish make-up | 3 |
| Completely unkempt, decorated, bizarre garments | 4 |

### 11. Insight

| | |
|---|---|
| Present, admits illness, agrees with need for treatment | 0 |
| Possibly ill | 1 |
| Admits behavior change, but denies illness | 2 |
| Admits possible changes in behavior, but denies illness | 3 |
| Denies any behavior change | 4 |

**Total score**                                                     .....

© Young RC, Biggs JT, Ziegler VT *et al*. **A rating scale for mania: reliability, validity and sensitivity.** *Br J Psychiatry* 1978; **133**:429–435.

# Assessment of hypomania

Hypomania may affect up to 50% of depressed patients [1]. However, it is frequently underdiagnosed in clinical practice, as there is a relative overdiagnosis of major depressive disorder at the expense of bipolar II disorder. It has been estimated that the correct diagnosis (and appropriate treatment) of patients with bipolar II disorder may be delayed by as many as 8–10 years [2,3].

All depressed patients should be screened for hypomania. DSM-IV and ICD-10 diagnostic criteria have been criticized for leading to underdiagnosis of hypomania because they lack sensitivity, particularly as they do not emphasize overactivity as a key diagnostic symptom, and require hypomanic symptoms to be present for a minimum of 4 days [4]. Furthermore, it has been proposed that hypomania should be added as a specifier to DSM-IV/ICD-10 diagnoses of a major depressive episode/disorder. Currently, major depression can be specified as catatonic, melancholic/ with somatic symptoms, atypical or post partum [5]. A hypomanic specifier would not necessitate the fulfilment of the criteria for a hypomanic or manic episode, but could consist merely of two or three symptoms of hypomania [6]. This amendment would help to increase the detection of bipolar II disorder in patients with major depression. Existing screening instruments (such as the Mood Disorder Questionnaire [MDQ]) are probably less sensitive at detecting bipolar II than bipolar I disorders [7].

Hypomania may occur as a single episode or as a continuous fluctuating state. The current theoretical perspective is that hypomania exists on a continuum from normal highs to mania [8,9]. The Hypomania Checklist (HCL) is based on this dimensional view. The instrument substantially reduces the proportion of false negatives arising from the Structured Clinical interview for DSM-IV (SCID) interview [6,10]. For example, a French version of the HCL increased the detection rate of bipolar II disorder from 22% with the SCID to 40% [11].

The HCL has recently been adapted into a 32-item self-administered questionnaire (HCL-32) to help identify the hypomanic component of depressive episodes and increase the detection rate of both bipolar II disorder and minor bipolar disorders (ie, hypomania accompanying dysthymia, minor depression or brief recurrent depression) [6].

# Featured scale

## Hypomania Checklist

The HCL-32 helps identify patients with bipolar II disorder who might otherwise be classified as suffering from a major depressive episode. It may also be useful in the identification of patients with minor bipolar disorders (eg, hypomanic symptoms in the presence of dysthymia, minor depression or recurrent brief depression). Because the HCL is self-administered by the patient, it has distinct advantages over lengthy structured interviews such as the SCID, and thus represents a useful tool for the busy clinician.

The HCL-32 comprises nine questions that assess:
- current mood state;
- usual mood state in comparison to others; and
- the characteristics of any 'high' periods including symptomatology, frequency, duration and social impact.

The questionnaire can usually be completed in 5–10 minutes.

Screening instruments require a higher sensitivity than specificity. The converse is true for diagnostic instruments. In a sample of outpatients with affective disorders, a cut-off score of 14 positive answers on the HCL-32 was associated with a sensitivity (true bipolars) of 80% and a specificity (true non-bipolars) of 51% for both bipolar I and bipolar II disorders [12].

The evaluation of the HCL is ongoing in multinational studies, but analyses consistently identify two factors – an 'advantageous' factor and a 'harmful' factor. The advantageous factor includes such symptoms as overactivity, elated mood and improved thinking, whereas the harmful factor includes risk-taking behavior, anger, irritability and flight of ideas. Similar factor structures were found in analyses of earlier versions of the HCL [13] and the MDQ [14], and also in a study of bipolar II patients who have remitted [15].

The self-assessment of hypomanic symptoms on the HCL-32 is not influenced by mood state [12]. Therefore, accurate self-reporting of hypomania appears to be feasible even in the presence of depression.

To test the use of the HCL-32 in nonclinical settings, Meyer et al. administered an online version of the checklist to 695 employees of a German university and a paper-and-pencil version to 408 Swedish individuals from a random sample from a representative population study [16]. While the Swedish results indicated a clear two-factor structure, the German data suggested a three-factor model [16]. Of the German participants, 11.1% reported hypomanic episodes lasting at least 4 days, versus 4.7% of the Swedish sample [16]. These individuals endorsed more HCL-32 symptoms than other participants and had higher rates of current and former depression and psychotherapy [16].

Another study used the HCL-32 to identify hypomanic features among 600 patients with bipolar I disorder and 322 major recurrent depressive disorder [17]. A cutoff score of 20 had the best combination of sensitivity and specificity for differentiating between bipolar I disorder and major depressive disorder, at 68% and 83%, respectively [17]. Interestingly, a score of 20 on the HCL-32 was recorded by 17% of major recurrent depressive disorder patients [17].

The HCL-32 has been developed in a range of languages and is currently undergoing validation. The Spanish version of the checklist was administered to 62 bipolar I disorder patients, 56 bipolar II disorder patients, 58 major depression patients, and 60 healthy controls on two occasions 4 weeks apart [18]. There were significant differences in the number of affirmative responses between the groups, at averages of 21.2, 19.3, 8.6, and 6.6 respectively [18]. The concurrent validity of the checklist was 0.72 and the test–retest reliability was 0.90 [18]. Using a cutoff of 14 affirmative responses, the HCL-32 had a sensitivity of 0.85 and a specificity of 0.79, while the positive and negative probability ratios were 4.1 and 5.3 [18].

Testing the Italian and Swedish versions of HCL-32, researchers administered the checklist to 266 bipolar disorder patients and 160 major depressive disorder patients from 186 Italian and 240 Swedish patients [19]. There were significant differences in HCL-32 scores between depression and bipolar disorder patients in both the Italian and Swedish groups, with both sets supporting a two factor structure of "active/ elevated" and "risk-taking/irritable" [19]. For the combined sample, a cutoff score of 14 or more yielded a sensitivity of 80%, a specificity of 51%, a positive predictive power of 73% and a negative predictive power of 61% [19]. A score of two or more on the "risk-taking/irritable" hypomania subscale had a sensitivity, specificity, positive predictive power and negative predictive power for recognising bipolar disorder of 76%, 62%, 76%, and 57%, respectively [19].

In another study of the Italian version of the HCL-32 of 123 patients referred to a tertiary care psychiatric division, 21.1% were diagnosed with bipolar or schizoaffective bipolar disorder, 58.8% with another Axis I disorder, and 41.24% were unaffected by any psychiatric disorder. The study revealed that the highest sensitivity (0.92) for the HCL-32 for identifying bipolar disorder was achieved using a cutoff score of 8, while the highest specificity, at 0.61, was seen with a cutoff score of 12 [20].

The same pattern was seen for the identification of bipolar II disorder, at a sensitivity of 0.90, and a specificity of 0.54 both for a cutoff score of 8 [20]. The researchers also found that the HCL-32 appeared to be more sensitive in detecting bipolar II disorder than the MDQ [20].

The Chinese version of the HCL-32 was tested in 199 psychiatric patients, of whom 66 had bipolar I disorder, 94 bipolar II disorder, and 39 major depression [21]. As with other versions of the HCL-32, a two-factor structure was identified [21]. At a cutoff score of 14, the sensitivity and specificity of the HCL-32 were 82% and 67%, respectively, while the positive and negative predictive values were 91% and 48%, respectively. The HCL-32 was also able to distinguish between bipolar I and II disorder using a cutoff score of 21, at a sensitivity of 64% and a specificity of 73% [21].

# HCL-32 Questionnaire

Rater: ....................................................................    Date: .......................................

## Patient's personal details

Name: ..............................................................    Age: ...........    Gender: M/F

## Energy, activity and mood

1) **First of all, how are you feeling today compared with your usual state:**
   *(Please mark only ONE of the following)*

   ☐ Much worse than usual          ☐ A little better than usual
   ☐ Worse than usual               ☐ Better than usual
   ☐ A little worse than usual      ☐ Much better than usual
   ☐ Neither better nor worse than usual

2) **How are you usually compared with other people?**
   Independently of how you feel today, please tell us how you are normally compared with other people, by marking which of the following statements describes you best.

   **Compared to other people my level of activity, energy and mood...**
   *(Please mark only ONE of the following)*

   ☐ ...is always rather stable and even    ☐ ...is generally lower
   ☐ ...is generally higher                 ☐ ...repeatedly shows periods of ups and downs

3) **Please try to remember a period when you were in a 'high' state.**
   How did you feel then? Please answer all these statements independently of your present condition.

   | **In such a state:** | **YES** | **NO** |
   |---|---|---|
   | 1. I need less sleep | ☐ | ☐ |
   | 2. I feel more energetic and more active | ☐ | ☐ |
   | 3. I am more self-confident | ☐ | ☐ |
   | 4. I enjoy my work more | ☐ | ☐ |
   | 5. I am more sociable (make more phone calls, go out more) | ☐ | ☐ |
   | 6. I want to travel and do travel more | ☐ | ☐ |
   | 7. I tend to drive faster or take more risks when driving | ☐ | ☐ |
   | 8. I spend more/too much money | ☐ | ☐ |
   | 9. I take more risks in my daily life (in my work and/or other activities) | ☐ | ☐ |

|  | YES | NO |
|---|---|---|
| 10. I am physically more active (sport, etc) | ☐ | ☐ |
| 11. I plan more activities or projects | ☐ | ☐ |
| 12. I have more ideas, I am more creative | ☐ | ☐ |
| 13. I am less shy or inhibited | ☐ | ☐ |
| 14. I wear more colourful and more extravagant clothes/make-up | ☐ | ☐ |
| 15. I want to meet or actually do meet more people | ☐ | ☐ |
| 16. I am more interested in sex and/or have increased sexual desire | ☐ | ☐ |
| 17. I am more flirtatious and/or am sexually more active | ☐ | ☐ |
| 18. I talk more | ☐ | ☐ |
| 19. I think faster | ☐ | ☐ |
| 20. I make more jokes or puns when I am talking | ☐ | ☐ |
| 21. I am more easily distracted | ☐ | ☐ |
| 22. I engage in lots of new things | ☐ | ☐ |
| 23. My thoughts jump from topic to topic | ☐ | ☐ |
| 24. I do things more quickly and/or more easily | ☐ | ☐ |
| 25. I am more impatient and/or get irritable more easily | ☐ | ☐ |
| 26. I can be exhausting or irritating for others | ☐ | ☐ |
| 27. I get into more quarrels | ☐ | ☐ |
| 28. My mood is higher, more optimistic | ☐ | ☐ |
| 29. I drink more coffee | ☐ | ☐ |
| 30. I smoke more cigarettes | ☐ | ☐ |
| 31. I drink more alcohol | ☐ | ☐ |
| 32. I take more drugs (sedatives, anxiolytics, stimulants, etc) | ☐ | ☐ |

**4)  Did the questions above, which characterize a 'high', describe how you are...**
*(Please mark only ONE of the following)*

... sometimes? ☐ → if you mark this box, please answer all of questions 5 to 9

... most of the time? ☐ → if you mark this box, please answer only questions 5 and 6

... I never experienced such a 'high' ☐ → if you mark this box, please stop here

**5)  Impact of your 'highs' on various aspects of your life:**

|  | Positive and negative | Positive | Negative | No impact |
|---|---|---|---|---|
| Family life | ☐ | ☐ | ☐ | ☐ |
| Social life | ☐ | ☐ | ☐ | ☐ |
| Work | ☐ | ☐ | ☐ | ☐ |
| Leisure | ☐ | ☐ | ☐ | ☐ |

6)  **Other people's reactions and comments to your 'highs'.**
    **How did other people close to you react to or comment on your 'highs'?**
    - ☐ Positively (encouraging or supportive)
    - ☐ Neutral
    - ☐ Negatively (concerned, annoyed, irritated, critical)
    - ☐ Positively and negatively
    - ☐ No reactions

7)  **Length of your 'highs' as a rule (on average):**
    *(Please mark only ONE of the following)*

    - ☐ 1 day
    - ☐ 2–3 days
    - ☐ 4–7 days

    - ☐ longer than 1 week
    - ☐ longer than 1 month
    - ☐ I can't judge/don't know

8)  **Have you experienced such 'highs' in the past 12 months?**
    - ☐ Yes
    - ☐ No

9)  **If yes, please estimate how many days you spent in 'highs' during the last 12 months:**
    Taking all together: about .............. days

© Angst J, Adolfsson R, Benazzi F *et al.* **The HCL-32: towards a self-assessment tool for hypomanic symptoms in outpatients.** *J Affect Disord,* 2005; **88**:217–233.

# Chapter 8

# Health-related quality of life assessment in bipolar disorder

The World Health Organization has identified bipolar disorder as the sixth leading cause of disability worldwide [1]. Bipolar disorder has a substantial impact on health-related quality of life (HRQoL), social and occupational functioning and work productivity. It also greatly increases healthcare utilization and costs. In fact, bipolar patients have been shown to utilize more healthcare services than patients with depression or chronic medical illnesses [2]. The direct cost of bipolar disorder in the United States (to which inpatient costs are the highest contributor) was estimated to be US$60 billion in 1999, with indirect costs estimated at almost US$30 billion [3].

In a recent review of HRQoL [2], patients with bipolar disorder were rated similarly in terms of HRQoL to patients with 'unipolar depression' (major depressive disorder), but equal to if not lower than patients with chronic medical illnesses. Furthermore, improvements in HRQoL scores take longer to be seen than symptomatic improvement [4] and there is evidence that, with recurrent bipolar episodes, progressive deterioration in functioning may occur [5,6]. With adequate containment of their disease, patients with bipolar disorder can improve their social and occupational functioning, sustain high work productivity and achieve acceptable HRQoL, which in turn should reduce service utilization and lifetime healthcare costs.

The assessment of HRQoL thus forms an important part of the evaluation of the individual with bipolar disorder. However, the complex nature of the disease, with symptomatic variation over relatively short periods of time, can complicate assessment. Various scales have been used to assess HRQoL in bipolar disorder and a few are discussed in this chapter.

## Briefly mentioned scales

### Medical Outcomes Study Core Survey Instrument
The Medical Outcomes Study (MOS) [7] was a 2-year study of patients with chronic medical conditions.

The Core Survey Instrument used to evaluate HRQoL in the MOS consists of 62 questions containing 116 items that assess a variety of different domains, namely:
- health and daily activities (three questions);
- physical health (six questions);
- pain (six questions);

- daily activities (four questions),
- feelings (38 questions);
- social activities (three questions);
- health (one question); and
- sleep (one question).

It is self-rated and takes about 30–60 minutes to complete. Scoring instructions and a user's manual are available, which describe the development of the measures, discuss their validity and reliability, and present psychometric results from the MOS.

## Medical Outcomes Study 20-Item Short-Form Health Survey

The 20-Item Short-Form Health Survey (SF-20) [8] is an abbreviated form of the 36-Item Short-Form Health Survey (SF-36), which in turn is a subset of the MOS Core Survey Instrument described above. The SF-20 has been further abbreviated to create the SF-12 and SF-8.

The SF-20 is self-rated but was designed to reduce the burden on the respondent while achieving minimum standards of precision in order to compare different groups on a variety of health dimensions. It takes about 3–5 minutes to complete, can be conducted via interview by telephone, and consists of six domains:
- physical functioning (six items);
- role functioning (two items);
- social functioning (one item);
- mental health (five items);
- current health perceptions (five items); and
- pain (one item).

## Quality of Life Index

The Quality of Life Index (QLI) [9] measures both satisfaction with various aspects of life and the importance of each of these aspects to the individual concerned. Thus, importance ratings are used to weight the satisfaction responses to give an individualized score [10].

The QLI is a two-part instrument:
- part 1 measures satisfaction on 33 items; and
- part 2 measures the importance of each item to the individual.

Scores are calculated for:
- quality of life overall;
- health and functioning;
- psychological/spiritual;

- social and economic; and
- family.

The QLI is a self-administered questionnaire that takes 10 minutes to complete. Scoring instructions are available at www.uic.edu/orgs/qli. It has well-established reliability, validity and sensitivity, and is available in a variety of different languages. Several versions of the QLI have been produced and used across a wide range of medical conditions. General population data are available for comparative purposes.

## 32-Item Behavioral and Symptom Identification Scale

The 32-item Behavioral and Symptom Identification Scale (BASIS-32) [11] is a self-report questionnaire that evaluates change in symptoms and problems over the course of treatment. It is typically administered at the time of a patient's admission and at discharge, and can be used for outpatient follow-up. It covers a wide spectrum of symptoms and diagnoses and has been validated in both inpatient and outpatient settings.

The scale consists of 32 items that measure the degree of difficulty experienced by the patient over the preceding week in relation to the following domains:
- relation to self and others;
- depression and anxiety;
- daily living and role functioning;
- impulsive and addictive behavior; and
- psychosis.

Each item is rated on a five-point scale ranging from no difficulty to extreme difficulty.

# Featured scale

## EQ-5D/EuroQol

The EQ-5D is commonly called the EuroQol [12,13] after the group who developed it. The multidisciplinary EuroQol group originally consisted of researchers from Europe, but membership is now international. The EQ-5D was developed as a standardized measure of health outcome across a range of health conditions and treatments. It provides a simple descriptive profile and a single index value for health status. These characteristics have made it a popular choice for use in population health surveys and in clinical and economic studies evaluating healthcare costs and utilization.

The EQ-5D is a self-report instrument consisting of two parts: a questionnaire (known as the descriptive system) and a visual analogue scale (VAS).

The descriptive system addresses the following five dimensions (hence 5D):
- mobility;
- self-care;
- usual activities;
- pain/discomfort; and
- anxiety/depression.

The responses on the five dimensions of the descriptive system give a unique EQ-5D health state. This information can be used as an EQ-5D health profile for individuals or groups, either at a single point or over a period of time. Differences in these profiles can be used to describe treatment outcomes. In addition, a weighted health state index can be derived from the EQ-5D using scores from 'value sets' elicited from general population samples. The EQ VAS consists of a vertically graduated VAS on which the respondent rates their self-rated health status. Scores on the VAS can be used in conjunction with the scores on the descriptive system to build a composite picture of an individual's state of health. Differences in this scale over time can be used as a measure of outcome. Thus, because of its simplicity, the EQ-5D takes only a few minutes to complete and is ideally suited for use in postal surveys as well as in clinics and face-to-face interviews. It is available in a number of different languages. Full details are available at www. euroqol.org.

The association between EQ-5D scores to current mood state in bipolar disorder was examined in 221 bipolar disorder patients from across the UK, of whom 51 were currently in a depressive episode and 21 in a hypomania/mania/mixed episode [14]. Scores on the ED-5Q were significantly, albeit moderately, correlated with scores on the Longitudinal Interval Follow-up Evaluation, the Hamilton Rating Scale for Depression, and the Beck Depression Inventory [14]. There were also significant differences in EQ-5D Index scores between the euthymic group (76 patients), the residual symptoms group (55 patients), the subsyndromal depressed group (40 patients), and the depressed subgroup (33 patients), at 1.00, 0.85, 0.81, and 0.41, respectively [14].

# EQ-5D/EuroQol

Rater: ................................................................    Date: .....................................

## Patient's personal details

Name: ................................................................    Age: ............    Gender: M/F

**Your own health state today**

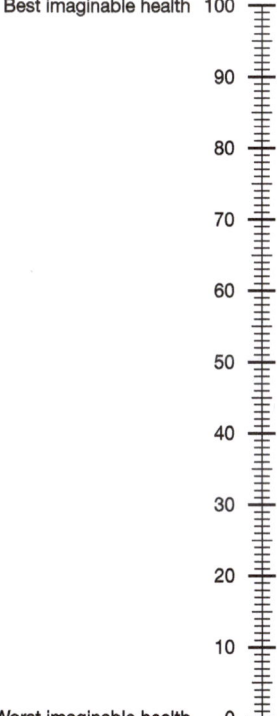

Best imaginable health  100

Worst imaginable health  0

# Chapter 9

# Assessment of pediatric bipolar disorder

Historically, bipolar disorder in children and adolescents has been grossly under-diagnosed. Epidemiological studies indicate that at least 20% of patients with bipolar disorder have their first episode before the age of 19 years [1,2]. A major clinical hurdle is the difficulty in accurately diagnosing bipolar disorder in this population and distinguishing it from other common psychiatric conditions, such as attention deficit hyperactivity disorder (ADHD) and conduct disorder (CD). Furthermore, a misdiagnosis of schizophrenia occurs frequently because of the high rate of psychotic symptoms in adolescents with bipolar disorder [3]. Variable presentation and lack of awareness of the condition also contribute to the under-diagnosis problem.

There are serious clinical implications for both false-negative and false-positive diagnoses in this group. Bipolar disorder is associated with profound academic impairment and social disability, with a significant risk of suicide [4]. Delayed recognition and treatment increases the risk of a more complicated course with more serious outcomes [5]. Furthermore, misdiagnosis of bipolar disorder as ADHD and treatment with neurostimulants can trigger manic episodes. Thus, false-negative diagnoses are costly events with grave implications for the patient and his/her family. Similarly, false-positive diagnoses of bipolar disorder and inappropriate treatment with anticonvulsants or lithium unnecessarily expose the patient to the potentially harmful side effects of these medications. Thus, there is a significant clinical need to detect and accurately diagnose bipolar disorder in children and adolescents. The various scales described below can assist the clinician in screening for the disorder, rating the overall severity of functional impairment and accurately distinguishing bipolar disorder from other psychiatric conditions frequently encountered in this age group.

## Briefly mentioned scales

### Child Behavior Checklist

The Child Behavior Checklist (CBCL) [6,7] is a screening instrument for emotional, behavioral and psychiatric problems as reported by parents. It is designed to assess in a standardized format the behavioral problems and social competencies of children and as such can be used as a useful screening instrument for bipolar disorder [8]. Various studies have demonstrated the checklist to have good validity and reliability [9]. In particular, many parents with bipolar disorder are concerned about the possibility that they may have passed on emotional problems to their children and the CBCL is a useful screening tool to address these concerns.

The checklist can be completed by the parents themselves or can be administered by a clinician during an interview with the parents.

It takes about 15 minutes to complete and consists of two sections:
• part 1 addresses the competence of the child (20 questions); and
• part 2 enquires about emotional and behavioral problems over the preceding 6 months (120 questions).

Parents rate their child for how true each item is using the following scale:
0 = *not true (as far as you know)*;
1 = *somewhat or sometimes true*;
2 = *very true or often true*.

The CBCL can be supplemented with information from Teacher Report Forms, Youth Self-Reports and Direct Observation Forms. The CBCL identifies emotional and behavioral problems in three general areas and eight specific areas.

The three general areas are:
• **internalizing problems:** inhibited or over-controlled behavior (eg, anxiety or depression);
• **externalizing problems:** antisocial or under-controlled behavior (eg, delinquency or aggression);
• **total problems:** all mental health problems reported by parents or adolescents.

The eight specific areas are:
• **somatic complaints:** chronic physical complaints without known cause or medically verified basis;
• **delinquent behavior:** breaking rules and norms set by parents and communities (eg, lying, swearing, stealing or truancy);
• **attention problems:** difficulty concentrating and sitting still, and impaired school performance;
• **aggressive behavior:** bullying, teasing, temper tantrums and fighting;
• **social problems:** impaired peer relationships;
• **withdrawn:** shyness and social isolation;
• **anxiety/depression:** feelings of loneliness, sadness, being unloved, worthlessness, anxiety and general fears;
• **social problems:** strange behavior or ideas, obsessions.

Although the CBCL has demonstrated some ability to discriminate between bipolar disorder and childhood disorders characterized by disruptive behavior, the CBCL does not formally assess manic or hypomanic symptoms. Instead, the high overall score generated by this instrument in children with bipolar disorder is due to high scores on subscales evaluating attention problems, aggression or anxiety/depression [10]. Thus, the CBCL is not specific for bipolar disorder and its discriminant ability is due to the fact that bipolar disorder in children typically involves greater symptom severity and functional impairment than other more common disorders of childhood.

When faced with a high score on the CBCL, clinicians must consider whether it represents bipolar disorder or a severe form of a more common condition (such as ADHD), or comorbidity of bipolar disorder and another condition. To help resolve such diagnostic dilemmas, more disease-specific scales should be employed, such as those discussed below.

Pediatric bipolar disorder, as diagnosed by the CBCL, occurs in approximately 1% of children [11,12]. A study of 5418, 3562, and 1971 Dutch twin pairs at ages 7, 10, and 12 indicated that the prevalence of CBCL-juvenile bipolar disorder phenotype was 0.8%, 0.9%, and 0.9%, respectively, in female participants and 0.8%, 0.9%, and 1.2% in male participants [11]. Furthermore, of the children with the CBCL-attention problems phenotype also met the criteria for the juvenile bipolar disorder phenotype [11]. In a separate study of 2856 children and adolescents aged 4–18 years, the 6-month prevalence of CBCL pediatric bipolar disorder was 0.7%. The subjects also had significantly greater social problems and delinquent behavior, higher suicidality rates, reduced need for sleep and hypersexual behavior compared with unaffected participants [12].

Nevertheless, the usefulness of the CBCL for identifying pediatric bipolar disorder remains controversial, with studies yielding conflicting results [13–15]. One assessment of data from two family studies of attention deficit hyperactivity disorder (ADHD) involving 471 probands and 410 siblings indicated a prevalence of lifetime bipolar disorder of 4.7% for probands and 3.4% for siblings, and 2.8% and 2.0%, respectively, for current bipolar disorder [13]. The area under the receiver operating characteristics curve (AUC) was 0.89 for probands and 0.85 for siblings, suggesting that the CBCL was a highly efficient method of detecting individuals with a lifetime history of pediatric bipolar disorder [13].

In contrast, a study of 1346 individuals from 657 complete and 32 incomplete twin pairs revealed that none of the 33 (2.5%) participants with CBCL juvenile bipolar disorder had a semi-structured interview diagnosis of DSM-IV bipolar disorder [14]. However, they were at significantly increased risk of suicidal behavior [14]. A study of 157 bipolar patients, 101 major depressive/anxiety disorder patients, 127 disruptive behavior disorder patients, and 128 healthy controls aged less than 12 years indicated that the sensitivity of CBCL pediatric bipolar disorder for identifying individuals with bipolar disorder was 57% and the specificity was 70–77% [15]. The

CBCL also had only moderate accuracy, at an AUC of 0.72–0.78, leading the researchers to conclude that the CBCL is not a useful proxy for a DSM-IV bipolar disorder diagnosis [15].

## Young Mania Rating Scale – Parent Version

The Young Mania Rating Scale – Parent Version (P-YMRS) [16] consists of 11 questions that parents are asked about their child's present mental state. It is usually completed in about 5–10 minutes. Like the adult scale (YMRS), seven items are rated on a scale of 0–4 and four are given additional weight (rated 0, 2, 4, 6 or 8). Thus, the maximum score is 60.

In one study, the average parental score in children with mania was 25 and with hypomania was 20, but there was frequent disagreement between the parent and clinician ratings [10]. A score above 13 was considered indicative of a potential case of mania or hypomania for the group that was studied, while a score above 21 was deemed a 'probable case'. A high score can help support a diagnosis in cases where there is a high risk (eg, both parents have bipolar disorder) but at the very least it suggests further diagnostic investigation should be undertaken (eg, with the featured scale discussed below), as the P-YMRS has a relatively high false-positive rate.

## Children's Global Assessment Scale

The Children's Global Assessment Scale (CGAS) [17] is an adaptation of the Global Assessment Scale for adults [18], which later became the GAF scale (*see* Chapter 2). The CGAS provides a measure of overall severity of disturbance. Such global assessment of functioning can help identify children in need of psychiatric treatment. It can also have predictive value and can measure change in functioning over time, therefore it may be particularly useful for monitoring the effects of therapeutic intervention.

The CGAS is a 100-point rating scale measuring psychological, social and school functioning for children aged 6–17 years. It is easy to use and contains operationalized anchor points for each decade of scores. It demonstrates both discriminant and concurrent validity, and good interrater reliability [19].

# Featured scale

## Washington University in St Louis Kiddie Schedule for Affective Disorders and Schizophrenia

The Washington University in St Louis Kiddie Schedule for Affective Disorders and Schizophrenia (WASH-U-KSADS) [20,21] was developed specifically to target the assessment of prepubertal mania and hypomania, to assess the pattern of rapid cycling and to generate diagnoses fulfilling DSM-IV criteria. It was considered particularly important to be able to identify and characterize comorbid ADHD, and to assess rapid cycling as this diagnosis occurs more frequently in child populations than in adult populations [22]. The scale is a modified version of the 1986 KSADS instrument [23] with expanded prepubertal mania and rapid cycling sections, and additional categories to include other DSM-IV diagnoses including ADHD. It demonstrates good validity [20], interrater reliability [21] and 6-month stability [24]. The WASH-U-KSADS is a semi-structured interview designed to assess children directly. It can be supplemented with interviews from the parents and by direct observation of the child. It should be administered by trained clinicians who have graduate degrees in psychiatry (or related fields) or who have appropriate postgraduate clinical experience. The interview takes a considerable amount of time to complete and is most useful for clinical research purposes.

# Washington University in St Louis Kiddie Schedule for Affective Disorders and Schizophrenia

Rater ................................................................    Date: .....................................

## Patient's personal details

Name: ................................................................    Age: ............    Gender: M/F

## 1. Elation, expansive mood

Elevated mood and/or optimistic attitude toward the future which lasted at least 4 hours and was out of proportion to the circumstances.

> Differentiate from normal mood in chronically depressed subjects. Do not rate positive if mild elation is reported in situations like Christmas gifts, birthdays, amusement parks, which normally overstimulate and make children very excited.

*Have (there been times when) you felt very good or too cheerful or high or terrific, great, or just not your normal self?*
    If unclear
    *When you felt on top of the world or as if there was nothing you couldn't do?*
    *...that this is the best of all possible worlds?*
    *Have you felt that everything would work out just the way you wanted?*
    *If people saw you, would they think you were just in a good mood or something more than that?*
    *Did you get as if you were drunk?*
    *Did you laugh a lot, get silly?*
    *Did you feel super-happy?*
    *When did this happen? (example)*

Coding instructions:

| | |
|---|---|
| No information | 0 |
| Not at all, normal, or depressed | 1 |
| Slight: good spirits, more cheerful than most people in his circumstances, but of only possible clinical significance | 2 |
| Mild: definitely elevated mood and optimistic outlook that is somewhat out of proportion to his circumstances | 3 |
| Moderate: mood and outlook are clearly out of proportion to circumstances, noticeable to others | 4 |
| Severe: quality of euphoric mood way out of proportion to circumstances | 5 |
| Extreme: clearly elated, almost constantly exalted expression, overexpansive | 6 |

**Rating:**    ____

Lifelong:

☐ yes          ☐ no

Only on follow-up assessments, show if onset was prior to rating period:

☐ yes          ☐ no

| | |
|---|---|
| Onset: age ............ years  ............ months | Onset: age ........... years   ............ months |
| date ............ month ............ year | date ........... month   ............ year |
| Onset: age ............ years  ............ months | Onset: age ........... years   ............ months |
| date ............ month ............ year | date ........... month   ............ year |
| Duration: ......... weeks | Duration: ......... weeks |
| ........... days (≥4 hours/day) per week | .......... days (≥4 hours/day) per week |

Be sure to use additional pages if there are more than two episodes

## 2. Decreased need for sleep

Less need for sleep than usual in order to feel rested (average for several days when needed less sleep). (Refer to norms on insomnia.)

*Have you needed less sleep than usual to feel rested?*

*How much sleep do you ordinarily need?*

*How much do you sleep when you are feeling so good?*

*When you wake up do you feel good and rested?*

*When you cannot fall asleep or when you get up through the night, what types of things do you do? Watch TV? Read? or do you do more active things? (eg, rearrange furniture? clean house? exercise?)*

*Do you have a lot of thoughts go through your mind when awake? What kinds of thoughts?*

*Do you worry? About what types of things?*

*How long are you awake for?*

*How often during the night? During the week?*

Coding instructions:

| | |
|---|---|
| No information | 0 |
| No change or more sleep needed | 1 |
| Up to 1 hour less than usual | 2 |
| Up to 2 hours less than usual | 3 |
| Up to 3 hours less than usual | 4 |
| Up to 4 hours less than usual | 5 |
| 4 or more hours less than usual | 6 |
| **Rating:** | —— |

Lifelong:

☐ yes          ☐ no

Only on follow-up assessments, show if onset was prior to rating period:

☐ yes          ☐ no

Onset: age ........... years ............ months        Onset: age ........... years ............ months
       date ........... month ............ year               date ........... month ............ year

Onset: age ........... years ............ months        Onset: age ........... years ............ months
       date ........... month ............ year               date ........... month ............ year

Duration: ......... weeks        Duration: ......... weeks

      .......... days (≥4 hours/day) per week              .......... days (≥4 hours/day) per week

---

Be sure to use additional pages if there are more than two episodes

---

## 3. Unusually energetic

More active than his usual level without expected fatigue.

*Have you had more energy than usual to do things?*
*Did people tell you that you were (are) non-stop?*
*Did you agree with them?*
*Did it seem like too much energy?*
*Do you know why?*
*Were you doing too many things?*
*Did you feel tired?*
*When did this happen? (example)*

Coding instructions:

| | |
|---|---|
| No information | 0 |
| No different than usual or less energetic | 1 |
| Slightly more energetic but of questionable significance | 2 |
| Little change in activity level but less fatigued than usual | 3 |
| Somewhat more active than usual with little or no fatigue | 4 |
| Much more active than usual with little or no fatigue | 5 |
| Unusually active all day long with little or no fatigue | 6 |
| **Rating:** | ___ |

Lifelong:

☐ yes          ☐ no

Only on follow-up assessments, show if onset was prior to rating period:

☐ yes          ☐ no

Onset: age ........... years ............ months        Onset: age ........... years ............ months
       date ........... month ............ year               date ........... month ............ year

Onset: age ........... years ............ months        Onset: age ........... years ............ months
       date ........... month ............ year               date ........... month ............ year

Duration: ......... weeks                     Duration: ......... weeks

.......... days (≥4 hours/day) per week       .......... days (≥4 hours/day) per week

Be sure to use additional pages if there are more than two episodes

## 4. Increase in goal-directed activity

As compared with usual level. Consider changes in scholastic, social, sexual, or leisure involvement or activity level associated with work, family, friends, new projects, interests or activities (eg, telephone calls, letter writing).

> *Is there any time when you were more active or involved in things compared to the way you usually are?*
> *What about in school, in your club, scouts, church, at home, friends, hobbies, new projects or interests?*
> *Were you doing a lot of things?*
> *How much of your day has been spent in this?*
> *Were you trying to do so many different things that you couldn't keep up?*
> *When did this happen? (example)*

Coding instructions:

| | |
|---|---|
| No information | 0 |
| No change or decrease | 1 |
| Slightly more interest or activity but of questionable significance | 2 |
| Mild but definite increase in general activity level involving several areas | 3 |
| Moderate generalized increase in activity level involving several areas | 4 |
| Marked increase and almost constantly involved in numerous activities in many areas | 5 |
| Extreme: eg, constantly active in a variety of activities from awakening till he goes to sleep | 6 |

**Rating:**

Lifelong:
☐ yes        ☐ no

Only on follow-up assessments, show if onset was prior to rating period:
☐ yes        ☐ no

Onset: age ........... years ............ months    Onset: age ........... years ............ months
       date ........... month ............ year              date ........... month ............ year

Onset: age ........... years ............ months    Onset: age ........... years ............ months
       date ........... month ............ year              date ........... month ............ year

Duration: ......... weeks                     Duration: ......... weeks

.......... days (≥4 hours/day) per week       .......... days (≥4 hours/day) per week

Be sure to use additional pages if there are more than two episodes

## 5. Grandiosity

Increased self-esteem and appraisal of his worth, power or knowledge (up to grandiose delusions) as compared with usual level. Persecutory delusions should not be considered evidence of grandiosity unless the subject feels the persecution is due to some special attributes of his (eg, power, knowledge).

*Have you felt more self-confident than usual?*
*Have you felt you are much better than others? smarter? stronger? Why?*
*Have you felt that you are a particularly important person or that you had special talents or abilities?*
*What about special plans?*
*When did this happen? (example)*

Useful enquiries to establish whether a grandiose delusion exists are: (1) *'How do you know?'* or an equivalent question to judge if the answer fits reality testing. For example, a mother reported that her obese, 10-year-old plain appearing child was planning to go to Hollywood to be an ultraslim model. The mother noted that the child was 'absolutely sure' that she could do this in spite of her physical appearance. (2) *'What does the child/adolescent do about the idea?'* For example, the child who wanted to be a model was on the Internet planning transportation to Hollywood. Another common example are children with high IQs who fail courses because they don't like their teacher. These children have the delusion that it is acceptable in our society for children to set the school rules. They act on their delusion by failing courses in which they usually get As and by calling school principals to complain about their teachers.

Coding instructions:

| | |
|---|---|
| No information | 0 |
| Not at all or decreased self-esteem | 1 |
| Slight: somewhat more confident about himself, but of doubtful clinical significance | 2 |
| Mild: definitely overestimates or exaggerates at least two of his talents, abilities, prospects or plans | 3 |
| Moderate: disproportionately inflated self-esteem involving several areas of functioning | 4 |
| Severe: marked, global, overevaluation of himself and his abilities, but falls short of true delusions | 5 |
| Extreme: clear grandiose delusions | 6 |

**Rating:**  ___

Lifelong:
☐ yes     ☐ no

Only on follow-up assessments, show if onset was prior to rating period:
☐ yes     ☐ no

Onset: age ........... years ........... months     Onset: age ........... years ........... months
       date ........... month ........... year               date ........... month ........... year

Onset: age ........... years ........... months     Onset: age ........... years ........... months date ............ month ............ year          date ........... month  ............ year

Duration: ......... weeks                          Duration: ......... weeks

.......... days (≥4 hours/day) per week          .......... days (≥4 hours/day) per week

Be sure to use additional pages if there are more than two episodes

## 6. Accelerated, pressured or increased amount of speech

*When you were (...) were there times that you spoke very rapidly or talked on and on and couldn't be stopped?*
*Did people say you were talking too much?*
*Could people understand you?*

Coding instructions:

| | |
|---|---|
| No information | 0 |
| Not at all or retarded speech | 1 |
| Slight increase which is of doubtful clinical significance | 2 |
| Mild: noticeably more verbose than normal but conversation is not strained | 3 |
| Moderate: so verbose that conversation is strained | 4 |
| Marked: so rapid that conversation is difficult to maintain | 5 |
| Extreme: talks rapidly or continuously and cannot be interrupted. Conversation extremely difficult or impossible | 6 |
| **Rating:** | |

Lifelong:

☐  yes          ☐  no

Only on follow-up assessments, show if onset was prior to rating period:

☐  yes          ☐  no

Onset: age ........... years  ............ months     Onset: age ........... years    ............ months
        date ........... month ............ year                date ........... month   ............ year

Onset: age ........... years  ............ months     Onset: age ........... years    ............ months
        date ........... month ............ year                date ........... month   ............ year

Duration: ......... weeks                          Duration: ......... weeks

.......... days (≥4 hours/day) per week          .......... days (≥4 hours/day) per week

Be sure to use additional pages if there are more than two episodes

## 7. Racing thoughts

Subjective experience that thinking was markedly accelerated.

*When you were (...) were there times when your thoughts raced through your mind?*
*Did you have more ideas than usual or more than you could handle?*

Coding instructions:

| | |
|---|---|
| No information | 0 |
| Not at all | 1 |
| Doubtful | 2 |
| Mild: occasional racing thoughts at least three times per week | 3 |
| Moderate: racing thoughts at least 50% of awake time | 4 |
| Severe: racing thoughts most of the time | 5 |
| Extreme: almost constant racing thoughts | 6 |
| **Rating:** | |

Lifelong:
☐ yes        ☐ no

Only on follow-up assessments, show if onset was prior to rating period:
☐ yes        ☐ no

Onset: age ............ years ............ months       Onset: age ........... years ............ months
       date ............ month ............ year                date .......... month ............ year

Onset: age ............ years ............ months       Onset: age ........... years ............ months
       date ............ month ............ year                date .......... month ............ year

Duration: ......... weeks                              Duration: ......... weeks

        .......... days (≥4 hours/day) per week                ......... days (≥4 hours/day) per week

Be sure to use additional pages if there are more than two episodes

## 8. Flight of ideas (observational or reported by informant)

Accelerated speech with abrupt changes from topic to topic usually based on understandable associations, distracting stimuli or play on words. In rating severity consider speed of associations, inability to complete ideas and sustain attention in a goal-directed manner. When severe, complete or partial sentences may be galloping on each other so fast that apparent sentence to sentence derailment and/or sentence incoherence may also be present. An extreme example of this symptom is 'You have to be quiet to be sad. Everything having to do with "s" is quiet – on the q.t. – sit, sob, sigh, sin, sorrow, surcease, sought, sand, sweet mother's love and salvation.'

*Have there been times when people could not understand you?*
*When they said you did not make sense?*
*Could you give me an example?*

Coding instructions:

| | |
|---|---|
| No information | 0 |
| Not at all or some other form of disturbances of thought or speech | 1 |
| Slight: occasional instances, which are of doubtful clinical significance | 2 |

| | |
|---|---|
| Mild: occasional instances of abrupt change in the topic with some impairment in understandability. More than 5% of sentence to sentence transitions are abrupt | 3 |
| Moderate: frequent instances with moderate impairment in understandability (>10%) | 4 |
| Severe: very frequent instances with definite impairment in understandability (>25%) | 5 |
| Extreme: most of speech consists of such rapid changes of topic that it is impossible to follow (>50%) | 6 |

**Rating:**

Lifelong:

☐ yes          ☐ no

Only on follow-up assessments, show if onset was prior to rating period:

☐ yes          ☐ no

Onset: age ............ years ............ months          Onset: age ........... years ............ months
         date ........... month ............ year                   date ........... month ............ year

Onset: age ............ years ............ months          Onset: age ........... years ............ months
         date ........... month ............ year                   date ........... month ............ year

Duration: ......... weeks          Duration: ......... weeks

         .......... days (≥4 hours/day) per week                   .......... days (≥4 hours/day) per week

Be sure to use additional pages if there are more than two episodes

## 9. Poor judgment

Excessive involvement in dangerous activities without recognizing the high potential for painful consequences.

> When you were (...), did you do anything that caused trouble for you or your family...or friends? What about anything that could have?
> Did you do things you normally wouldn't do (like giving away a whole lot of things or taking a whole lot of chances)?
> Did you think of what would happen before you did it?
> Was there anything that you did that you now think you should not have done?
> Do you like to talk on the phone? How often do you talk on the phone? What time of day or night? Whom do you call? Do you ever call stars or famous people you admire? Do you call 900 numbers or long distance? What are the charges on the phone bills?
> Are you friendly to people you just met? Do you talk to them on the phone? Take them home?
> Do you like to shop or buy things? Ever order from catalogues? TV shopping? Join CD, video, or book clubs? Buy or order things you don't really need? Give your friends expensive gifts or your belongings? How do you pay for these things?
> Do you ever play games for money or belongings? Make bets? Gamble?
> What about take dares from others? Are you a risk-taker?

Coding instructions:

| | |
|---|---|
| No information | 0 |
| Not at all | 1 |
| Slight: Of doubtful clinical significance | 2 |
| Mild: eg, calls friends at odd hours | 3 |
| Moderate: eg, purchases many things he doesn't need and can't afford or gives money away | 4 |
| Severe: eg, on impulse, goes to places without plans or money and takes too many chances | 5 |
| Very severe: attempts activities with potentially very dangerous consequences | 6 |

**Rating:** ___

Lifelong:

☐ yes        ☐ no

Only on follow-up assessments, show if onset was prior to rating period:

☐ yes        ☐ no

Onset: age ............ years ............ months        Onset: age ........... years ............ months
       date ............ month ............ year                date ........... month ............ year

Onset: age ............ years ............ months        Onset: age ........... years ............ months
       date ............ month ............ year                date ........... month ............ year

Duration: ......... weeks                               Duration: ......... weeks

       .......... days (≥4 hours/day) per week                  .......... days (≥4 hours/day) per week

Be sure to use additional pages if there are more than two episodes

## 10. Distractibility (observational or reported by informant)

Child presents evidence of difficulty focusing his attention on the questions of the interviewer, jumps from one thing to another, cannot keep track of his/her answers, and is drawn by irrelevant stimuli he cannot shut off. Not to be confused with avoidance of uncomfortable themes.

*Have you ever been told that you have trouble sticking to what you are supposed to do? Did you? Can you give me an example? Has a teacher told you that you 'always' get distracted?*

Coding instructions:

| | |
|---|---|
| No information | 0 |
| Not at all | 1 |
| Slight: of doubtful clinical significance | 2 |
| Mild: present but responds to structuring and repetition | 3 |

| | |
|---|---|
| Moderate: difficult to complete interview because of child's inattentiveness which doesn't respond to structure | 4 |
| Severe: impossible to complete interview because of child's inattentiveness | 5 |
| **Rating:** | |

Lifelong:
☐ yes        ☐ no

Only on follow-up assessments, show if onset was prior to rating period:
☐ yes        ☐ no

Onset: age ........... years ............ months        Onset: age ........... years    ........... months
         date ........... month ............ year                 date ........... month    ........... year

Onset: age ........... years ............ months        Onset: age ........... years    ........... months
         date ........... month ............ year                 date ........... month    ........... year

Duration: ......... weeks        Duration: ......... weeks

          ........... days (≥4 hours/day) per week                  ........... days (≥4 hours/day) per week

> Be sure to use additional pages if there are more than two episodes

> Note: If any of the prior items or irritability is positive, establish the chronology and determine if they occurred simultaneously. The rest of the questions in this section should be directed to such period(s) of time. If none of the above is positive ask the following items anyway for any period of time during the current episode.

## 11. Motor hyperactivity

Visible manifestations of generalized motor hyperactivity which occurred during a period of abnormally elevated, expansive, or irritable period. Make certain that the hyperactivity actually occurred and was not merely a subjective feeling of restlessness. Make certain this is not chronic but episodic hyperactivity.

> *When you were (...), were there times when you were (high, feeling so good, so angry) that you were always moving, could not stay put, were unable to sit still or you always had to be moving, pacing up and down? Or are you always like that?*

Coding instructions:

| | |
|---|---|
| No information | 0 |
| Not at all or retarded | 1 |
| Slight increase which is of doubtful clinical significance | 2 |
| Mild: unable to sit quietly in a chair | 3 |
| Moderate: paces about a great deal | 4 |
| Marked: almost constantly moving and pacing about | 5 |
| Extreme: so hyperactive that he would exhaust himself if not restrained | 6 |
| **Rating:** | |

Lifelong:

☐  yes          ☐  no

Only on follow-up assessments, show if onset was prior to rating period:

☐  yes          ☐  no

Onset: age ........... years ............ months     Onset: age ........... years     ............ months
       date ........... month ............ year                date ........... month    ............ year

Onset: age ........... years ............ months     Onset: age ........... years     ............ months
       date ........... month ............ year                date ........... month    ............ year

Duration: ......... weeks                            Duration: ......... weeks

........... days (≥4 hours/day) per week                    ........... days (≥4 hours/day) per week

Be sure to use additional pages if there are more than two episodes

Note: Documentation for motor hyperactivity and psychomotor agitation can be similar. During a period of abnormally elevated, expansive or irritable mood has any of the following occurred?

## 12. Inappropriate laughing, joking, or grinning

*Do you sometimes laugh or act silly? Does this happen for no reason? Do other people notice? Do you laugh out loud in class? Are the other students quietly doing their work? Do you sometimes act or talk like a much younger child? Do you use baby talk? Do you ever crawl like a baby?*

Coding instructions:

| | |
|---|---|
| No information | 0 |
| Not at all: laughter appropriate to situation | 1 |
| Slight: occasional inappropriate laughter of doubtful significance | 2 |
| Mild: eg, child receives verbal reprimands from teacher for laughing in class three times in one week | 3 |
| Moderate to severe: eg, child sent to principal's office or given detention three times or more in one week | 4 |

**Rating:** ___

Lifelong:

☐  yes          ☐  no

Only on follow-up assessments, show if onset was prior to rating period:

☐  yes          ☐  no

Onset: age ........... years ............ months     Onset: age ........... years     ............ months
       date ........... month ............ year                date ........... month    ............ year

Onset: age ........... years ............ months     Onset: age ........... years     ............ months
       date ........... month ............ year                date ........... month    ............ year

Duration: ......... weeks                           Duration: ......... weeks

  .......... days (≥4 hours/day) per week            .......... days (≥4 hours/day) per week

Be sure to use additional pages if there are more than two episodes

## 13. Uninhibited people seeking, gregariousness

*Do you like meeting new people? Are you friendly with people you just met? Do your parents ever complain that you are always bringing new people home? How often does this happen? Do you find yourself bringing home 'friends' that your parents have never seen before? How often does this happen?*

*Do people comment that you are 'the most popular' person at the party?*

*Do you begin conversations with people you have never met? (eg, at the mall do you go up and talk to just anyone)? Are you the type of person who never met a 'stranger'?*

*Are you the 'class clown'?*

Coding instructions:

| | |
|---|---|
| No information | 0 |
| Not at all or shy | 1 |
| Doubtful: occasionally more talkative or social | 2 |
| Mild: definitely present (eg, parent reprimands child three times in one week for talking to strangers) | 3 |
| Moderate to severe: eg, child puts self in danger, cannot be left unsupervised for fear that the child will leave with strangers; adolescent brings home new acquaintances once a week | 4 |

**Rating:**                                                                      ____

Lifelong:

☐ yes        ☐ no

Only on follow-up assessments, show if onset was prior to rating period:

☐ yes        ☐ no

Onset: age ............ years ............ months    Onset: age ........... years   ............ months
         date ........... month ............ year                 date ........... month   ............ year

Onset: age ........... years ............ months    Onset: age ........... years   ............ months
         date ........... month ............ year                 date ........... month   ............ year

Duration: ......... weeks                           Duration: ......... weeks

  .......... days (≥4 hours/day) per week            .......... days (≥4 hours/day) per week

Be sure to use additional pages if there are more than two episodes

## 14. Increased productivity

*Are there times when you start many more projects than you could possibly complete in an hour's time (eg, go to music lesson, rearrange your bedroom, play two different sports, start an art project)?*
*Are there times when you feel that you have to produce more than anyone else (eg, sell 100 times more Girl Scout cookies than anyone else)?*

Coding instructions:

| | |
|---|---|
| No information | 0 |
| Not at all – or decreased | 1 |
| Doubtful: may start two projects at one time | 2 |
| Mild: definitely more productive or initiates several projects at the same time | 3 |
| Moderate to severe: initiates many projects at the same time with unrealistic or unobtainable goals within the time allotted. Won't stop projects to eat or sleep | 4 |

**Rating:**

Lifelong:
☐ yes        ☐ no

Only on follow-up assessments, show if onset was prior to rating period:
☐ yes        ☐ no

Onset: age ........... years ............ months        Onset: age ........... years ............ months
          date ........... month ............ year                    date ........... month ............ year

Onset: age ........... years ............ months        Onset: age ........... years ............ months
          date ........... month ............ year                    date ........... month ............ year

Duration: ......... weeks                              Duration: ......... weeks

          ........... days (≥4 hours/day) per week              .......... days (≥4 hours/day) per week

Be sure to use additional pages if there are more than two episodes

## 15. Sharpened and unusually creative thinking

*Do you like to write stories, do art projects, draw, play music, or write songs? Do you feel that you are 'outstanding' at these activities when you're feeling high? Are there times when you feel that you are 'super' creative?*

Coding instructions:

| | |
|---|---|
| No information | 0 |
| Not at all – average creativity | 1 |
| Doubtful: occasionally shows more creativity than usual, but of doubtful significance | 2 |
| Mild: definitely present. Spends more time on creative activities (eg, writing, drawing, etc) | 3 |

Moderate to severe: able to produce imaginative stories, songs, plays or art work of better than individual's usual quality in a short time span

4
___

**Rating:**

___

Lifelong:

☐ yes          ☐ no

Only on follow-up assessments, show if onset was prior to rating period:

☐ yes          ☐ no

| | |
|---|---|
| Onset: age ........... years ............ months | Onset: age .......... years ............ months |
| date ........... month ............ year | date .......... month ............ year |
| Onset: age ........... years ............ months | Onset: age .......... years ............ months |
| date ........... month ............ year | date .......... month ............ year |
| Duration: ......... weeks | Duration: ......... weeks |
| .......... days (≥4 hours/day) per week | .......... days (≥4 hours/day) per week |

Be sure to use additional pages if there are more than two episodes

## 16. Hypersexuality

**Parent of child 6–12 years:**

*Are there times when your child makes inappropriate sexual remarks to a teacher or adult? Does your child like to 'talk dirty' (eg, talk about private parts of the body inappropriately)? Do adults complain that your child touches breasts or other private areas? When at the store does your child have to look at 'Playboy' magazines? Does your child search out books or magazines with nude or suggestive pictures? Does your child draw naked people?*

**Child 6–12 years:**

*What magazines do you like at the store? What type of movies do you like to watch? What kind of pictures do you draw?*

Observe child for sexually explicit language or behavior during the interview (eg, trying to touch interviewer's body; propositioning the interviewer; talking about seeing sex).

**Adolescents:**

*Are there times when you have to have sex no matter what time of day it is? Are there times when there are not enough sexual partners to meet your needs? Are there times when there are not enough hours in the day to have as much sex as you want and need? Do you talk nonstop about your many sexual conquests? Do you call the sex hotline and run up high phone bills?*

Be sure to distinguish this behavior from provocation to sexual activity in the environment (eg, see the sexual abuse section of the Psychosocial Schedule for School-Age Children).

Coding instructions:

| | |
|---|---|
| No information | 0 |
| Not at all | 1 |

| | |
|---|---|
| Doubtful: occasional sexual comment or gesture | 2 |
| Mild: makes inappropriate explicit sexual comments, drawings or gestures one time a week | 3 |
| Moderate to severe: overt sexual behaviors or language occurs multiple times each week or at inappropriate times. Major episode one time a week (eg, adolescent sleeps with three partners at the same time). | 4 |

**Rating:** ___

Lifelong:
☐ yes      ☐ no

Only on follow-up assessments, show if onset was prior to rating period:
☐ yes      ☐ no

Onset: age ........... years ............ months    Onset: age ........... years ............ months
       date ........... month ............ year             date ........... month ............ year

Onset: age ........... years ............ months    Onset: age ........... years ............ months
       date ........... month ............ year             date ........... month ............ year

Duration: ......... weeks                          Duration: ......... weeks
       ........... days (≥4 hours/day) per week             ........... days (≥4 hours/day) per week

Be sure to use additional pages if there are more than two episodes

## 17. Influence of illicit drugs or alcohol on onset of 'high' periods.

*A lot of kids use drugs or alcohol. Do you? Can you remember times when you felt high and you were not drinking or using drugs?*

Coding instructions:

| | |
|---|---|
| N/A or no information. | 0 |
| Never under the influence of alcohol or drugs, or no mania present | 1 |
| Sometimes but not always under the influence of alcohol or drugs At least once he was manic or hypomanic without prior drug or alcohol use | 2 |
| Only under the influence of alcohol or drugs | 3 |

**Rating:** ___

Lifelong:
☐ yes      ☐ no

Only on follow-up assessments, show if onset was prior to rating period:
☐ yes      ☐ no

Onset: age ........... years ............ months    Onset: age ........... years ............ months
       date ........... month ............ year             date ........... month ............ year

Onset: age ........... years ............ months    Onset: age ........... years ............ months date ............ month ............ year         date ........... month ............ year

Duration: ......... weeks                 Duration: ......... weeks

........... days (≥4 hours/day) per week     .......... days (≥4 hours/day) per week

Be sure to use additional pages if there are more than two episodes

## 18. Number and duration of manic and hypomanic episode item

Rater should record the number of episodes lasting the specified period of time during the rating period.

1. <1 day        ..................
2. 1–2 days      ..................
3. 2–3 days      ..................
4. 3–6 days      ..................
5. 7–13 days    ..................
6. ≥14 days      ..................

Has there ever been a time when you/your child/adolescent continuously or almost continuously cycles?

☐ yes        ☐ no

Does it appear that you/your child/adolescent has multiple cycles in a single day?

☐ yes        ☐ no

What is the largest number of cycles you/your child/adolescent has in a day?

Write in number     ................

When you/your child/adolescent continuously or almost continuously cycles which pattern or patterns occur?

a. Changing (going) from high to even moods    ☐ yes    ☐ no

b. Changing (going) from high to low moods     ☐ yes    ☐ no

c. Having a mixture of high, low and even moods ☐ yes    ☐ no

Note: If the mood is described as irritable, write in detail the sequence of moods (eg, high to low to irritable). For some subjects, it will be possible to determine if the irritable mood is also high or low; for other subjects this may not be possible. Describe in detail what activities and thoughts and other feelings accompany the irritable mood.

What age were you/your child/adolescent when continuous or almost continuous cycling first appeared?

Write in age     ................

Onset and offset of periods of continuous or almost continuous cycling:

Lifelong:

☐  yes          ☐  no

Only on follow-up assessments, show if onset was prior to rating period:

☐  yes          ☐  no

Onset: age ........... years ........... months          Onset: age ........... years ........... months
       date ........... month ........... year                 date ........... month ........... year

Onset: age ........... years ........... months          Onset: age ........... years ........... months
       date ........... month ........... year                 date ........... month ........... year

Duration: ......... weeks          Duration: ......... weeks

      .......... days (≥4 hours/day) per week                .......... days (≥4 hours/day) per week

Be sure to use additional pages if there are more than two episodes

© Geller B, Zimerman B, Williams M *et al.* Reliability of the Washington University in St. Louis Kiddie Schedule for Affective Disorders and Schizophrenia (WASH-U-KSADS) mania and rapid cycling sections. *J Am Acad Child Adolesc Psychiatry* 2001; **40**:450–455.

# Chapter 10

# Assessment of comorbidities

Bipolar disorder is associated with a high rate of psychiatric comorbidity [1], with one analysis of European data indicating that up to 75% of patients with any bipolar disorder have at least one DSM-IV comorbidity [2]. The most common comorbid conditions include substance use disorders, anxiety disorders, eating disorders and personality disorders [3–5]. The association between bipolar disorder and eating disorders has been shown in several epidemiological studies [6–8]. More than 10% of bipolar patients may have eating disorders. Conversely, in patients with anorexia or bulimia, the lifetime prevalence of bipolar disorder is between 4% and 6% [9]. However, although the disordered eating behaviors reported by many bipolar patients are problematic, they do not fulfil the criteria for a specific eating disorder.

Seasonal variation in mood is well recognized in patients with affective disorders [10], particularly bipolar disorder [11]. Carbohydrate craving and increased food intake are typical of winter depressions (seen commonly in type II bipolar disorder and four times more frequently in women than men) [12]. Binge eating is observed more commonly among bipolar patients than in the general population. In one study, 38% of bipolar patients exhibited full or partial binge eating disorders [13]. This is characterized by the intake of large amounts of food in the absence of hunger, and associated with a subjective sense of lack of control; eating more rapidly than usual until feeling uncomfortably full; feeling disgusted, depressed or guilty after each binge; and concern for the long-term effects on weight and body image. To fulfil DSM-IV-R criteria, binges should occur on average at least 2 days per week for at least 6 months.

Bipolar disorder is associated with obesity (21–32%) and being overweight (58%) [14–17]. Beyond eating disorders, the causes include subclinical hypothyroidism (related to treatment with lithium carbonate), inactivity and drug-related obesity. Obesity is a common side effect of treatment with olanzapine, clozapine, valproate and lithium [18–20]. In addition, drugs associated with dry mouth (eg, anticholinergics) can also lead to weight increase through increased drinking to ease the symptom, particularly of high-calorie drinks.

Obesity is associated with a myriad of complications, both physical (cardiovascular disease, type 2 diabetes) and psychological (poor self-image, low self-esteem), which diminish overall quality of life and reduce longevity. Obesity has also been associated with poor outcome in bipolar disorder [21]. There is a need to develop clinical strategies to monitor, prevent and ameliorate obesity and weight gain in patients with bipolar disorder. Such strategies need to reflect the broad range of causes and diverse symptomatology and provide management programmes tailored to the individual.

The Barcelona Bipolar Eating Disorder Scale (BEDS) was developed to detect and quantify disordered eating behavior in bipolar patients.

## Featured scale

### Barcelona Bipolar Eating Disorder Scale

The BEDS quantifies disordered eating behavior in bipolar patients [20]. It rapidly and effectively evaluates both the severity and frequency of maladaptive eating behaviors. Such assessment enables treatment strategies to be tailored to individual patient needs.

The BEDS is a simple, 10-item, self-administered scale that usually takes 1–2 minutes to complete. Each item can be scored from 0 (never) to 3 (always), allowing for a maximum score of 30 in total.

The BEDS explores disturbed eating patterns under the following general headings:
• regularity of eating;
• influence of mood state on eating patterns;
• binge eating and night eating;
• influence of fullness on eating;
• compulsive eating; and
• carbohydrate craving.

The design of the BEDS scale drew on items from pre-existing eating scales, and also from specific complaints regarding their eating habits from a group of 350 bipolar patients interviewed by the authors. A committee of experts selected the 10 most relevant and independent items. The clinical cut-off score was estimated from the median score of a sample of 55 healthy controls plus two standard deviations. The median score was 6 (mean 6.6) with a standard deviation of 3.7. Thus, a cut-off score of 13 was selected. Patients scoring above 13 may require individualized intervention to evaluate and manage their eating disturbances.

A validation study of the BEDS was conducted in 90 patients diagnosed with bipolar disorder and eating disturbances, followed-up for 6 months, and 40 healthy controls [20]. The researchers found that the scale had adequate feasibility, at a non-response rate of less than 2.5% [20]. The internal consistency was high for patients, at a Cronbachs alpha coefficient of 0.79, but was lower for controls, at a coefficient of 0.57 [20]. The BEDS had an acceptable ability to discriminate between patients and controls, at an area under the receiver operating characteristics curve of 0.85 [20]. The scale also had moderate correlation with the Bulimic Investigatory Test Edinburgh, at an $r$ value of 0.32–0.64, but low correlations with the Barratt Impulsiveness Scale, the Young Mania Rating Scale, and the Hamilton Depression Rating Scale 17, at r values less than 0.3 [20].

# Barcelona Bipolar Eating Disorder Scale

Rater: ............................................................... Date: .....................................

## Patient's personal details

Name: ............................................................... Age: ............ Gender: M/F

|  | 0 | 1 | 2 | 3 |
|---|---|---|---|---|
| 1. Do you find it difficult to follow the schedules for the different meals regularly without missing any of them? | ☐ | ☐ | ☐ | ☐ |
| 2. Do you believe that your mood state plays a role in having more or less appetite? | ☐ | ☐ | ☐ | ☐ |
| 3. Have you ever needed to get up in the night in order to eat? | ☐ | ☐ | ☐ | ☐ |
| 4. Do you find it difficult to stop eating when you want to even though you are full? | ☐ | ☐ | ☐ | ☐ |
| 5. Do you tend to eat more when you are depressed? | ☐ | ☐ | ☐ | ☐ |
| 6. If you are euphoric, does your appetite change? | ☐ | ☐ | ☐ | ☐ |
| 7. Do you sometimes have eating binges, with the sensation of not being able to stop eating? | ☐ | ☐ | ☐ | ☐ |
| 8. Would you say you tend to eat sweets? | ☐ | ☐ | ☐ | ☐ |
| 9. Do you consider that you generally have too great an appetite and eat excessively? | ☐ | ☐ | ☐ | ☐ |
| 10. Do you tend to eat between meals? | ☐ | ☐ | ☐ | ☐ |

**Total** ......................

© Torrent C, Vieta E, Crespo J et al. **Barcelona Bipolar Eating Disorder Scale (BEDS): a self-administered scale for eating disturbances in bipolar patients.** Actas Esp Psiquiatr 2004; **32**:127–131.

# Chapter 11

# Assessment of functioning

Bipolar disorder patients have high rates of psychosocial morbidity that commonly affects independent living, and vocational and social activities, which is exacerbated by the early onset of the disease [1,2]. In one study of 53 patients who recently experienced their first mania episode with or without psychosis, 62.3% met the criteria for full remission of mood symptoms. Yet, the same proportion of patients was found to have at least moderate functional disability [2]. At 6-months follow-up, 25.7% of patients had at least moderate disability, and better functioning at 6 months was associated with remission of depressive symptoms [2]. A European analysis suggested that only approximately 70% of bipolar disorder patients are either unemployed or receive disability payments [3].

The association between functional impairment and employment status in bipolar disorder was examined in a study involving 213 veterans with bipolar disorder, of whom 91 were employed [4]. The results indicated that neurocognitive function is significantly associated with employment [4]. In addition, the findings demonstrated that employment status was significantly associated with lifetime psychiatric hospitalizations and the number of psychotropic medications prescribed [4].

It has been shown that, over a relatively short follow-up, functional impairment may predict subsequent depressive symptoms [5]. For the analysis, 92 bipolar I disorder patients were assessed at baseline and after 4 months, which revealed moderate functional impairment at both timepoints. Although functioning at baseline was not linked to manic symptoms at 4 months, depressive symptom levels at follow-up were associated with baseline functioning [5].

In order to assess the functioning difficulties experienced by psychiatric patients, particularly bipolar disorder patients, the Functioning Assessment Short test (FAST) was developed.

## Featured scale

### Functioning Assessment Short Test (FAST)

The FAST assesses functional impairment, focusing on the primary problems experienced by the mentally ill, including bipolar disorder patients [1].

The FAST is a simple, easy-to-use, 24-item, clinician-administered scale that is designed to take a short time to complete [1]. Specifically, it refers to the last 15 days before assessment [1].

Each item is rated on a 4-point scale [1]:
0 = no difficulty
1 = mild difficulty
2 = moderate difficulty
3 = severe difficulty

The global score is obtained when the scores from each item are added, with a higher score indicating greater disability [1].

The items are divided into six areas of functioning [1]:
- autonomy;
- occupational functioning;
- cognitive functioning;
- financial issues;
- interpersonal relationships; and
- leisure time.

The validity and reliability of the FAST was assessed in 101 patients with bipolar disorder and 61 healthy controls [1]. All items of the FAST were answered by 99% of the patients in every test session, and the average time spent completing the instrument was 6.00 minutes [1]. The average FAST score for patients was 25.43, while that for controls was 6.0 [1]. The scale had high internal consistency, at a Cronbach's alpha coefficient of 0.909 [1]. The area under the receiver operating characteristics curve for discriminating between patients and controls was 0.86 [1]. Using a cutoff score of 11, the FAST has a sensitivity and specificity of 72% and 87% respectively [1]. FAST scores were significantly lower in euthymic patients than in manic and depressed patients, at respective scores of 18.55, 40.44, and 43.21 [1].

# Functioning Assessment Short Test

Rater: ...................................................    Date: ....................................

## Patient's personal details

Name: ...............................................    Age: ............    Gender: M/F

> **Guide for scoring items:**
>
> To what extent is the patient experiencing difficulties in the following aspects? Ask the patient about the areas of difficulty in functioning and score according to the following scale: (0): no difficulty, (1): mild difficulty, (2): moderate difficulty, (3): severe difficulty.

**Autonomy**

1. Taking responsibility for a household       0 ☐    1 ☐    2 ☐    3 ☐
2. Living on your own                          0 ☐    1 ☐    2 ☐    3 ☐
3. Doing the shopping                          0 ☐    1 ☐    2 ☐    3 ☐
4. Taking care of yourself (physical aspects, hygiene)    0 ☐    1 ☐    2 ☐    3 ☐

**Occupational functioning**

5. Holding down a paid job                     0 ☐    1 ☐    2 ☐    3 ☐
6. Accomplishing tasks as quickly as necessary    0 ☐    1 ☐    2 ☐    3 ☐
7. Working in the field in which you were educated    0 ☐    1 ☐    2 ☐    3 ☐
8. Occupational earnings                       0 ☐    1 ☐    2 ☐    3 ☐
9. Managing the expected work load             0 ☐    1 ☐    2 ☐    3 ☐

**Cognitive functioning**

10. Ability to concentrate on a book, film     0 ☐    1 ☐    2 ☐    3 ☐
11. Ability to make mental calculations        0 ☐    1 ☐    2 ☐    3 ☐
12. Ability to solve a problem adequately      0 ☐    1 ☐    2 ☐    3 ☐
13. Ability to remember newly-learned names    0 ☐    1 ☐    2 ☐    3 ☐
14. Ability to learn new information           0 ☐    1 ☐    2 ☐    3 ☐

**Financial issues**

15. Managing your own money                    0 ☐    1 ☐    2 ☐    3 ☐
16. Spending money in a balanced way           0 ☐    1 ☐    2 ☐    3 ☐

**Interpersonal relationships**

17. Maintaining a friendship or friendships           0 ☐   1 ☐   2 ☐   3 ☐

18. Participating in social activities                0 ☐   1 ☐   2 ☐   3 ☐

19. Having good relationships with people close you   0 ☐   1 ☐   2 ☐   3 ☐

20. Living together with your family                  0 ☐   1 ☐   2 ☐   3 ☐

21. Having satisfactory sexual relationships          0 ☐   1 ☐   2 ☐   3 ☐

22. Being able to defend your interests               0 ☐   1 ☐   2 ☐   3 ☐

**Leisure time**

23. Doing exercise or participating in sport          0 ☐   1 ☐   2 ☐   3 ☐

24. Having hobbies or personal interests              0 ☐   1 ☐   2 ☐   3 ☐

# Chapter 12

# Assessment of suicidality

Suicide and suicidality among patients with bipolar disorder are important public health concerns. It is estimated that between 21% and 54% of bipolar disorder patients will attempt suicide [1].

Furthermore, bipolar disorder patients have markedly increased rates of suicide death [2]. A UK study involving 46,136 patients with severe mental illness and 300,426 unaffected patients attending 755 general practices revealed that, compared with unaffected individuals, bipolar disorder patients had hazard ratios for suicide death of 14.2, 14.8, and 24.8 at ages 18–30 years, 30–49 years, and 50–70 years, respectively [2].

Analysis of Finnish data on suicidal ideation among 90 bipolar I disorder and 101 bipolar II disorder patients indicated that levels of suicidal ideation are significantly higher in depressive, depressive mixed, and mixed phases, with no attempts made during hypomanic/manic phases [3]. In addition, levels of suicidal ideation were significantly correlated with levels of anxiety, hopelessness, and subjective and objective depression [3].

In another study, the same researchers found in a sample of 81 bipolar I disorder and 95 bipolar II disorder patients followed-up for 18 months that, compared with other phases, the incidence of suicide attempts was 37-fold higher during combined mixed and depressive mixed phases, and 18-fold higher during major depressive episodes [4].

There have been several studies examining demographic and clinical predictors of suicide attempt and death in bipolar disorder patients. In a US study of 32,360 individuals treated for bipolar disorder at two large prepaid health plans, men were found to have a significantly lower rate of suicide than women, but a higher rate of suicide death, at respective hazard ratios of 0.68 and 2.70 [5]. Suicide attempt, but not suicide death, was significantly associated with substance use comorbidity, at a hazard ratio of 2.53, while comorbid anxiety disorder was associated with an increased risk of both suicide attempt and death, at hazard ratios of 1.40 and 1.81, respectively [5].

It is therefore crucial that the risk of suicide in an individual with bipolar disorder be assessed.

# Featured scale

## Columbia Classification Algorithm of Suicide Assessment (C-CASA)

The C-CASA is a classification system for suicidality that incorporates definitions derived from empirical findings on suicidality and predictive and risk factors [6].

The C-CASA has eight categories that distinguish suicidal events from non-suicidal, indeterminate, or potentially suicidal events [6]:
• completed suicide;
• suicide attempt;
• preparatory acts towards imminent suicidal behavior;
• suicidal ideation;
• self-injurous behavior, no suicidal intent;
• other, no deliberate self-harm;
• self-injurous behavior, suicidal intent unknown; and
• not enough information.

Each category is accompanied by a definition and training examples that are designed to help the rater assign each act or event to the appropriate category [6].

In order to test the C-CASA, the system was applied to adverse event reports from 25 trials of antidepressant medications (24 sponsored by pharmaceutical companies) with a combined sample of 4562 pediatric patients aged 6–17 years treated between 1983 and 2004 [6]. All of the information was provided by the US Food and Drug Administration and assessed by nine internationally recognized expert raters, with events randomly assigned and each assessed by three raters [6].

The C-CASA rated 8.4% events as suicide attempt, 1.9% as preparatory acts toward imminent suicidal behavior, 14.5% as suicidal ideation, 8.2% as self-injurous behavior, suicidal intent unknown, 2.1% as not enough information, 4.0% as self-injurous behavior, no suicidal intent, and 60.9% as other, no deliberate self-harm [6]. The C-CASA had excellent overall reliability, at a median intraclass coefficient of 0.89 [6]. There was unanimous agreement between the three raters on 85.7% of events, agreement between two rates on 13.8% of events, and no agreement on 0.47% of events [6].

There was discrepancy between C-CASA ratings and pharmaceutical company ratings on 38 cases, 26 of which were new, possibly suicidal cases and 12 of which were previously labelled as suicidal but eliminated on the C-CASA [6]. There was relatively low agreement between C-CASA ratings and pharmaceutical ratings for the label "suicide attempt", with 57.7% of attempts identified by pharmaceutical companies downgraded by the C-CASA [6].

## Seriousness of disease

| Classification/Category | Definition | Training Examples |
|---|---|---|
| **Suicidal events** | | |
| Completed suicide | A self-injurious behavior that resulted in fatality and was associated with at least some intent to die as a result of the act | 1) After a long argument with his girlfriend, which resulted in the end of their relationship, the patient collected a rope and rode his bike to an isolated area where he fatally hanged himself. A suicide note was later found<br><br>2) After four documented attempts at suicide, the patient stole his uncle's gun and shot himself and was fatally injured |
| Suicide attempt | A potentially self-injurious behavior, associated with at least some intent to die, as a result of the act.<br><br>Evidence that the individual intended to kill him/herself, at least to some degree, can be explicit or inferred from the behavior or circumstance. A suicide attempt may or may not result in actual injury. | 1) After a fight with her friends at school, in which they discontinued speaking with her, the patient ingested approximately 16 aspirin and eight other pills of different types on the school grounds. She said that she deserved to die, which was why she swallowed the pills<br><br>2) The patient used a razor blade to lacerate his wrists, his antecubital fossae, and his back bilaterally. He told his therapist that the "the main objective was to stop feeling like that," and he knew that he could die but didn't care. According to the patient, he also ingested a bottle of rubbing alcohol because in his health class he heard "that the medulla will get more suppressed that way," thereby increasing the chances that he would be "successful" and die |
| Preparatory acts toward imminent suicidal behavior | The individual takes steps to injure him- or herself, but is stopped by self or others from starting the self-injurious act before the potential for harm has begun | 1) The patient had run away from home overnight because his father had gone to school and retrieved a recent "bad" report card. He was fearful of his father's reaction. Upon his return home, a 5- to 6-hour argument with his parents ensued, and he took a vegetable (broad, sharp) knife and went to his room. He reported putting the knife to his wrist but never puncturing the skin<br><br>2) The patient stated that he "couldn't stand being depressed anymore" and "wanted to die." He decided to hang himself. He tied a telephone cord to the door knob and placed the cord loosely around his neck. Then, he stopped himself and did not follow through with the attempt |
| Suicidal ideation | Passive thoughts about wanting to be dead or active thoughts about killing oneself, not accompanied by preparatory behavior. | 1) Active: the patient reported to the doctor that he was thinking about hanging himself in the closet. He was taken to the hospital and admitted<br><br>2) Passive: the patient reported ideas about wanting to be dead but denied acting on these feelings |

## Seriousness of disease (Continued)

### Nonsuicidal events

| Self-injurious behavior, no suicidal intent | Self-injurious behavior associated with no intent to die. The behavior is intended purely for other reasons, either to relieve distress (often referred to as "self-mutilation," eg, superficial cuts or scratches, hitting/banging, or burns) or to effect change in others or the environment | 1) The patient was feeling ignored. She went into the family kitchen where her mother and sister were talking. She took a knife out of the drawer and made a cut on her arm. She denied that she wanted to die at all ("not even a little"), but she just wanted them to pay attention to her<br><br>2) The patient reported feeling agitated and anxious after a fight with her parents. She went into her room, locked the door, and made several superficial cuts on the inside of her arms. She stated that she felt relieved after cutting herself and that she did not want to die. She reported that she had done this before at times of distress and that it usually helped her feel better<br><br>3) The patient was in class, where a test was about to begin, and stabbed himself with a pencil in order to be taken to the nurse's office<br><br>4) A 14-year-old girl wrote her name on her arm with a penknife and said that she often does so in order to reduce her anxiety<br><br>5) The patient was noted to have multiple superficial burns on his arms. Upon questioning, he denied trying to kill himself |
|---|---|---|
| Other, no deliberate self-harm | No evidence of any suicidality or deliberate self-injurious behavior associated with the event. The event is characterized as an accidental injury, psychiatric or behavioral symptoms only, or medical symptoms or procedure only | 1) The patient had a cut on the neck from shaving<br><br>2) The patient was hospitalized for worsening of OCD or depressive symptoms with no suicidal thoughts or actions ;or<br><br>3) aggressive behavior<br><br>4) Hospitalization was because of an infection, hinoplasty, or pregnancy |

### Indeterminate or potentially suicidal events

| Self-injurious behavior, suicidal intent unknown | Self-injurious behavior where associated intent to die is unknown and cannot be inferred. The injury or potential for injury is clear, but why the individual engaged in that behavior is unclear | 1) The patient cut her wrists after an argument with her boyfriend<br><br>2) The patient was angry at her husband. She took 10–15 diazepam tablets and flushed the rest down the toilet. Her husband called the police for help, and she was taken to the hospital. She was groggy and stayed overnight in the hospital<br><br>3) A 9-year-old patient had spoken about suicide frequently. After learning that his baseball coach was retiring, he began scratching his arm with a pencil |
|---|---|---|

## Seriousness of disease (Continued)

| | | |
|---|---|---|
| Not enough information, insufficient information to determine whether the event involved deliberate suicidal behavior or ideation would warrant placement in this category | There is reason to suspect the possibility of suicidality but not enough to be confident that the event was not something other, such as an accident or psychiatric symptom. An injury sustained on a place on the body consistent with deliberate self-harm or suicidal behavior (eg, wrists), without any information as to how the injury was received | 1) A child who "stabbed himself in [the] neck with a pencil." The event may have been deliberate as opposed to accidental, as suggested by "stabbed," but not enough information was provided to determine whether the event was deliberate.<br><br>2) A cut on the neck |

# References

## Chapter 2: Global assessment scales

1.  Rush AJ, Kupfer DJ. Strategies and tactics in the treatment of depression. In: Treatments of Psychiatric Disorders, 2nd edn, Volume 1. Edited by GO Gabbard. Washington, DC: American Psychiatric Press, Inc., 1995; 1349–1368.

2.  Knopman DS, Knapp MJ, Gracon SI, et al. The Clinician Interview-Based Impression (CIBI): a clinician's global change rating scale in Alzheimer's disease. Neurology 1994; 44:2315–21.

3.  Lehmann E. Practicable and valid approach to evaluate the efficacy of nootropic drugs by means of rating scales. Pharmacopsychiatrie 1984; 17:71–5.

4.  Guy W. Clinical Global Impressions (CGI). In: ECDEU Assessment Manual for Psychopharmacology, revised. Rockville, MD: US Department of Health, Education and Welfare, NIMH, 1976;217–22.

5.  American Psychiatric Association. Diagnostic and Statistical Manual of Mental Disorders, 4th edn revised. Washington, DC: American Psychiatric Association, 2000.

6.  Luborsky L. Clinicians' judgement of mental health. Arch Gen Psychiatry 1962; 7:407–17.

7.  Endicott J, Spitzer RL, Fleiss JL, et al. The Global Assessment Scale: a procedure for measuring overall severity of psychiatric disturbance. Arch Gen Psychiatry 1976; 33:766–71.

8.  Goldman HH, Skodol AE, Lave TR. Revising axis V for DSM-IV: a review of measures of social functioning. Am J Psychiatry 1992; 149:1148–56.

9.  Altshuler LL, Gitlin MJ, Mintz J, et al. Subsyndromal depression is associated with functional impairment in patients with bipolar disorder. J Clin Psychiatry 2002; 63:807–11.

10. Martinez-Arán A, Vieta E, Colom F, et al. Cognitive impairment in euthymic bipolar patients: implications for clinical and functional outcome. Bipolar Disord 2004; 6:224–32.

11. Spearing MK, Post RM, Leverich GS, et al. Modification of the Clinical Global Impressions (CGI) scale for use in bipolar illness (BP): the CGI-BP. Psychiatry Res 1997; 73:159–71.

12. Beneke M, Rasmus W. 'Clinical global impressions' (ECDEU): some critical comments. Pharmacopsychiatry 1992; 25:171–6.

13. Vieta E, Torrent C, Martinez-Arán A, et al. A user-friendly scale for the short and long term outcome of bipolar disorder: the CGI-BP-M. Actas Esp Psiquiatr 2002; 30:301–4.

14. Dahlke F, Lohaus A, Gutzmann H. Reliability and clinical concepts underlying global judgments in dementia: implications for clinical research. Psychopharmacol Bull 1992; 28:425–32.

15. Weitkunat R, Letzel H, Kanowski S. Clinical and psychometric evaluation of the efficacy of nootropic drugs: characteristics of several procedures. Zeitschrift fiir Gerontopsychologie undpsychiatrie 1993; 6:51–60.

16. Vieta E, Parramon G, Padrell E, et al. Quetiapine in the treatment of rapid cycling bipolar disorder. Bipolar Disord 2002; 4:335–40.

17. Vieta E, Reinares M, Corbella B, et al. Olanzapine as long-term adjunctive therapy in treatment-resistant bipolar disorder. J Clin Psychopharmacol 2001; 21:469–73.

## Chapter 3: Detection of bipolar I

1.  Kessler RC, McGonagle KA, Zhao S, et al. Lifetime and 12-month prevalence of DSM-III-R psychiatric disorders in the United States: results from the National Comorbidity Survey. Arch Gen Psychiatry 1994; 51:8–19.

2.  Akiskal HS, Bourgeois ML, Angst J, et al. Re-evaluating the prevalence of and diagnostic composition within the broad clinical spectrum of bipolar disorders. J Affect Disord 2000; 59:S5–S30.

3.  Fajutrao L, Locklear J, Priaulx J, et al. A systematic review of the evidence of the burden of bipolar disorder in Europe. Clin Pract Epidemol Ment Health 2009; 5:3.

4.  Angst J. The emerging epidemiology of hypomania and bipolar II disorder. J Affect Disord 1998; 50:143–51.

5.  Judd LL, Akiskal HS. The prevalence and disability of bipolar spectrum disorders in the US population: re-analysis of the ECA database taking into account subthreshold cases. J Affect Disord 2003; 73:123–31.

6.  Hirschfeld RM, Lewis L, Vornik LA. Perceptions and impact of bipolar disorder: how far have we really come? Results of the National Depressive and Manic–Depressive Association 2000 survey of individuals with bipolar disorder. J Clin Psychiatry 2003; 64:161–74.

7.  Baca–Garcia E, Perez-Rodriguez MM, Basurte-Villamor I, et al. Diagnostic stability of psychiatric disorders in clinical practice. Br J Psychiatry 2007; 190:210–6.

8.  Salvatore P, Baldessarini RJ, Tohen M, et al. McLean-Harvard International first-episode project: two-year stability of DSM-IV diagnoses in 500 first-year episode psychotic disorder patients. J Clin Psychiatry 2009; 70:458–66.

9.  Perugi G, Micheli C, Akiskal HS, et al. Polarity of the first episode, clinical characteristics, and course of manic depressive illness: a systematic retrospective investigation of 320 bipolar I patients. Compr Psychiatry 2000; 41:13–8.

10.  Bowden CL. Strategies to reduce misdiagnosis of bipolar depression. Psychiatr Serv 2001; 52:51–5.

11.  Ghaemi SN, Sachs GS, Chiou AM, et al. Is bipolar disorder still underdiagnosed? Are antidepressants overutilized? J Affect Disord 1999; 52:135–44.

12.  Altshuler LL, Post RM, Leverich GS, et al. Antidepressant-induced mania and cycle acceleration: a controversy revisited. Am J Psychiatry 1995; 152:1130–8.

13.  Ghaemi SN, Boiman EE, Goodwin FK. Diagnosing bipolar disorder and the effect of antidepressants: a naturalistic study. J Clin Psychiatry 2000; 61:804–8.

14.  Hirschfeld RMA, Bowden CL, Perlis RH, et al. Practice guideline for the treatment of patients with bipolar disorder (revision). Am J Psychiatry 2002; 159:1–50.

15.  Swann AC, Bowden CL, Calabrese JR, et al. Differential effect of number of previous episodes of affective disorder on response to lithium or divalproex in acute mania. Am J Psychiatry 1999; 156:1264–6.

16.  Tondo L, Baldessarini RJ. Reduced suicide risk during lithium maintenance treatment. J Clin Psychiatry 2000; 61:97–104.

17.  Geller B, Cooper TB, Sun K, et al. Double-blind and placebo-controlled study of lithium for adolescent bipolar disorders with secondary substance dependency. J Am Acad Child Adolesc Psychiatry 1998; 37:171–8.

18.  FDA Public Health Advisory. Worsening Depression and Suicidality in Patients Being Treated with Antidepressant Medications. March 22, 2004; available online at www.fda.gov/cder/drug/antidepressants.

19.  Piver A, Yatham LN, Lam RW. Bipolar spectrum disorders. New perspectives. Can Fam Physician 2002; 48:896–904.

20. Manning JS, Haykal RF, Connor PD, et al. On the nature of depressive and anxious states in a family practice setting: the high prevalence of bipolar II and related disorders in a cohort followed longitudinally. Compr Psychiatry 1997; 38:102–8.

21. Glick ID. Undiagnosed bipolar disorder: new syndromes and new treatments. Prim Care Companion J Clin Psychiatry 2004; 6:27–33.

22. Ghaemi SN, Hsu DJ, Ko JY, et al. Bipolar spectrum disorder: a pilot study. Psychopathology 2004; 37:222–6.

23. Hirschfeld RMA, Williams JB, Spitzer RL, et al. Development and validation of a screening instrument for bipolar spectrum disorder: the Mood Disorder Questionnaire. Am J Psychiatry 2000; 157:1873–5.

24. Hirschfeld RMA, Holzer C, Calabrese JR, et al. Validity of the Mood Disorder Questionnaire: a general population study. Am J Psychiatry 2003; 160:178–180.

25. Miller CJ, Klugman J, Berv DA, et al. Sensitivity and specificity of the Mood Disorder Questionnaire for detecting bipolar disorder. J Affect Disord 2004; 81:167–71.

26. Twiss J, Jones S, Anderson I. Validation of the Mood Disorder Questionnaire for screening for bipolar disorder in a UK sample. J Affect Disord 2008; 110:180–4.

27. Weber Rouget B, Gervasoni N, Dubuis V, et al. Screening for bipolar disorders using a French version of the Mood Disorder Questionnaire (MDQ). J Affect Disord 2005; 88:103–8.

28. Gervasoni N, Weber Rouget B, Miguez M, et al. Performance of the Mood Disorder Questionnaire (MDQ) according to bipolar subtype and symptom severity. Eur Psychiatry 2009; in press.

29. Sanchez-Moreno J, Villagran JM, Gutierrez JR, et al. Adaptation and validation of the Spanish version of the Mood Disorder Questionnaire for the detection of bipolar disorder. Bipolar Disord 2008; 10:400–12.

30. Tafalla M, Sanchez-Moreno J, Diez T, et al. Screening for bipolar disorder in a Spanish sample of outpatients with current major depressive episode. Affect Disord 2009; 114:299–304.

31. Isometsä E, Suominen K, Mantere O, et al. The Mood Disorder Questionnaire improves recognition of bipolar disorder in psychiatric care. BMC Psychiatry 2003; 3:8.

32. Chung KF, Tso KC, Cheung E, et al. Validation of the Chinese version of the Mood Disorder Questionnaire in a psychiatric population in Hong Kong. Psychiatry Clin Neurosci 2008; 62: 464–71.

33. Konuk N, Kiran S, Tamam L, et al. [Validation of the Turkish version of the mood disorder questionnaire for screening bipolar disorders]. Turk Psikiyatri Derg 2007; 18:147–54.

34. Shabani A, Koohi-Habibi L, Nojomi M, et al. The persian bipolar spectrum diagnostic scale and mood disorder questionnaire in screening the patients with bipolar disorder. Arch Iran Med 2009; 12:41–7.

## Chapter 4: Detection of bipolar II

1. Vieta E, Gasto C, Otero A, et al. Differential features between bipolar I and bipolar II disorder. Compr Psychiatry 1997; 30:98–101.

2. American Psychiatric Association. Diagnostic and Statistical Manual of Mental Disorders, 4th edn revised. Washington, DC: American Psychiatric Association, 2000.

3. Angst J. The emerging epidemiology of hypomania and bipolar II disorder. J Affect Disord 1998; 50:143–51.

4.  Hirschfeld RM. Bipolar spectrum disorder: improving its recognition and diagnosis. J Clin Psychiatry 2001; 62:5–9.

5.  Manning JS. The Mood Disorder Questionnaire in primary care: (not) ready for prime time? Primary Care Companion J Clin Psychiatry 2002; 4:7–8.

6.  Vieta E, Suppes T. Bipolar II disorder: arguments for and against a distinct entity. Bipolar Disord 2008; 10:163–78.

7.  Pies R. Bipolar Spectrum Diagnostic Scale validation study. Paper presented at: American Psychiatric Association 155th Annual Meeting, Philadelphia, PA, USA; May 18–23, 2002.

8.  Miller CJ, Ghaemi SN, Klugman J, et al. Utility of mood disorder questionnaire and bipolar spectrum diagnostic scale. Program and abstracts of the American Psychiatric Association 155th Annual Meeting, Philadelphia, PA, USA; May 18–23, 2002 (Abstract NR2).

9.  Nassir Ghaemi S, Miller CJ, Berv DA, et al. Sensitivity and specificity of a new bipolar spectrum diagnostic scale. J Affect Disord 2005; 84:273–7.

10. Shabani A, Koohi-Habibi L, Nojomi M, et al. The Persian bipolar spectrum diagnostic scale and mood disorder questionnaire in screening the patients with bipolar disorder. Arch Iran Med 2009; 12:41–7.

## Chapter 5: Assessment of depression in bipolar disorder

1.  Perugi G, Micheli C, Akiskal HS, et al. Polarity of the first episode, clinical characteristics, and course of manic depressive illness: a systematic retrospective investigation of 320 bipolar I patients. Compr Psychiatry 2000; 41:13–8.

2.  Judd LL, Akiskal HS, Schettler PJ, et al. The long-term natural history of the weekly symptomatic status of bipolar I disorder. Arch Gen Psychiatry 2002; 59:530–7.

3.  Judd LL, Akiskal HS, Schettler PJ, et al. A prospective investigation of the natural history of the long-term weekly symptomatic status of bipolar II disorder. Arch Gen Psychiatry 2003; 60:261–9.

4.  Beck AT, Ward CH, Mendelson M, et al. An inventory for measuring depression. Arch Gen Psychiatry 1961; 4:561–71.

5.  Demyttenaere K, De Fruyt J. Getting what you ask for: on the selectivity of depression rating scales. Psychother Psychosom 2003; 72:61–70.

6.  Snaith P. Depression: detection and diagnosis. Br J Psychiatry 2002; 181:165.

7.  Richter P, Werner J, Heerlein A, et al. On the validity of the Beck Depression Inventory. A review. Psychopathology 1998; 31:160–8.

8.  Kumar G, Rissmiller DJ, Steer RA, et al. Mean Beck Depression Inventory-II total scores by type of bipolar episode. Psychol Rep 2006; 98:836–40.

9.  Montgomery SA, Asberg M. A new depression scale designed to be sensitive to change. Br J Psychiatry 1979; 134:382–9.

10. Snaith RP, Harrop FM, Newby DA, et al. Grade scores of the Montgomery-Asberg Depression and the Clinical Anxiety Scales. Br J Psychiatry 1986; 148:599–601.

## Chapter 6: Assessment of mania in bipolar disorder

1.  Diagnostic and Statistical Manual of Mental Disorders. 4th edition (revised). Washington, DC: American Psychiatric Association; 2000.

2.  World Health Organization. The ICD-10 Classification of Mental and Behavioral Disorders: Clinical Descriptions and Diagnostic Guidelines. Geneva, Switzerland: World Health Organization, 1992.

3. Poolsup N, Li Wan Po A, Oyebode F. Measuring mania and critical appraisal of rating scales. J Clin Pharm Ther 1999; 24:433–43.

4. Altman EG, Hedeker DR, Janicak PG, et al. The Clinician-Administered Rating Scale for Mania (CARS-M): development, reliability and validity. Biol Psychiatry 1994; 36:124–34.

5. Tohen M, Goldberg JF, Gonzalez-Pinto Arrillaga AM, et al. A 12-week, double-blind comparison of olanzapine vs haloperidol in the treatment of acute mania. Arch Gen Psychiatry 2003; 60:1218–26.

6. Chengappa KN, Baker RW, Shao L, et al. Rates of response, euthymia and remission in two placebo-controlled olanzapine trials for bipolar mania. Bipolar Disord 2003; 5:1–5.

7. Vieta E, Calabrese JR, Hennen J, et al. Comparison of rapid-cycling and non-rapid-cycling bipolar I manic patients during treatment with olanzapine: analysis of pooled data. J Clin Psychiatry 2004; 65:1420–8.

8. Young RC, Biggs JT, Ziegler VT, et al. A rating scale for mania: reliability, validity and sensitivity. Br J Psychiatry 1978; 133:429–435.

## Chapter 7: Assessment of hypomania

1. Angst J, Gamma A. A new bipolar spectrum concept: a brief review. Bipolar Disord 2002; 4:11–4.

2. Lish JD, Dime-Meenan S, Whybrow PC, et al. The National Depressive and Manic-Depressive Association (DMDA) survey of bipolar members. J Affect Disord 1994; 31:281–94.

3. Hirschfeld RMA, Calabrese JR, Weissman MM, et al. Screening for bipolar disorder in the community. J Clin Psychiatry 2003; 64:53–9.

4. Akiskal H, Bourgeois ML, Angst J, et al. Re-evaluating the prevalence of and diagnostic composition within the broad clinical spectrum of bipolar disorders. J Affect Disord 2000; 59:S5–S30.

5. Angst J, Gamma A, Benazzi F, et al. Diagnostic issues in bipolar disorder. Eur Neuropsychopharmacol 2003; 13:S43–S50.

6. Angst J, Gamma A, Benazzi F, et al. Towards a re-definition of subthreshold bipolarity: diagnosis and epidemiology of bipolar-II, minor bipolar disorders and hypomania. J Affect Disord 2003; 73:133–46.

7. Zimmermann M, Posternak MA, Chelminski I, et al. Using questionnaires to screen for psychiatric disorders: a comment on a study of screening for bipolar disorder in the community. J Clin Psychiatry 2004; 65:605–10.

8. Angst J. Categorical and dimensional perspectives of depression. In: Depressive Disorders, Volume 1. Edited by M Maj, N Sartorius. Chichester, New York, Weinheim: John Wiley & Sons, 1999; 54–6.

9. Korszun A, Moskvina V, Brewster S, et al. Familiality of symptom dimensions in depression. Arch Gen Psychiatry 2004; 61:468–74.

10. Benazzi F. Improving the mood disorder questionnaire to detect bipolar II disorder. Can J Psychiatry 2003; 48:770–1.

11. Allilaire J-F, Hantouche E-G, Sechter D, et al. Fréquence et aspects cliniques du trouble bipolaire II dans une étude multicentrique française: EPIDEP. Encéphale 2001; 27:149–58.

12. Angst J, Adolfsson R, Benazzi F, et al. The HCL-32: towards a self-assessment tool for hypomanic symptoms in outpatients. J Affect Disord, 2005; 88:217–33.

13. Hantouche EG, Angst J, Akiskal HS. Factor structure of hypomania: interrelationships with cyclothymia and the soft bipolar spectrum. J Affect Disord 2003; 73:39–47.

14. Benazzi F, Akiskal HS. The dual factor structure of self-rated MDQ hypomania: energized-activity versus irritable-thought racing. J Affect Disord 2003; 73:59–64.

15. Benazzi F. Toward better probing for hypomania of bipolar II disorder by using Angst's checklist. Int J Meth Psychiatr Res 2004; 13:1–9.

16. Meyer TD, Hammelstein P, Nilsson LG, et al. The Hypomania Checklist (HCL-32): its facto-rial structure and association to indices of impairment in German and Swedish nonclinical samples. Compr Psychiatry 2007; 48:79–87.

17. Forty L, Smith D, Jones L, et al. Identifying hypomanic features in major depressive disorder using the hypomania checklist (HCL-32). J Affect Disord 2009; 114:68–73.

18. Vieta E, Sanchez-Moreno J, Bulbena A, et al. Cross validation with the mood disorder questionnaire (MDQ) of an instrument for the detection of hypomania in Spanish: the 32 item hypomania symptom check list (HCL-32). J Affect Disord 2007; 101:43–55.

19. Angst J, Adolfsson R, Benazzi F, et al. The HCL-32: towards a self-assessment tool for hypomanic symptoms in outpatients. J Affect Disord 2005; 88:217–33.

20. Carta MG, Hardoy MC, Cadeddu M, et al. The accuracy of the Italian version of the Hypomania Checklist (HCL-32) for the screening of bipolar disorders and comparison with the Mood Disorder Questionnaire (MDQ) in a clinical sample. Clin Pract Epidemol Ment Health 2006; 2:2.

21. Wu YS, Angst J, Ou CS, et al. Validation of the Chinese version of the hypomania checklist (HCL-32) as an instrument for detecting hypo(mania) in patients with mood disorders. J Affect Disord 2008; 106:133–43.

## Chapter 8: Health-related quality of life assessment in bipolar disorder

1. Murray CJ, Lopez AD, Jamison DT. The global burden of disease in 1990: summary results, sensitivity analysis and future directions. Bull World Health Org 1994; 72:495–509.

2. Dean BB, Gerner D, Gerner RH. A systematic review evaluating health-related quality of life, work impairment, and healthcare costs and utilization in bipolar disorder. Curr Med Res Opin 2004; 20:139–154.

3. Wyatt RJ, Henter I. An economic evaluation of manic-depressive illness – 1991. Soc Psychiatry Psychiatr Epidemiol 1995; 30:213–19.

4. Dion GL, Tohen M, Anthony WA, et al. Symptoms and functioning of patients with bipolar disorder six months after hospitalization. Hosp Community Psychiatry 1988; 39:652–57.

5. Martinez-Arán A, Vieta E, Colom F, et al. Cognitive impairment in euthymic bipolar patients: implications for clinical and functional outcome. Bipolar Disord 2004; 6:224–32.

6. Keck PE, McElroy SL, Strakowski SM, et al. Outcome and comorbidity in first- compared with multiple-episode mania. J Nerv Ment Dis 1995; 183:320–4.

7. Stewart AL, Hays RD, Ware JE. Health perceptions, energy/fatigue, and health distress measures. In: Measuring Functioning and Well-Being: The Medical Outcomes Study Approach. Edited by AL Stewart, JE Ware. Durham, NC: Duke University Press, 1992; 143–72.

8. Ware JE, Sherbourne CD, Davies AR. Developing and testing the MOS 20-item short-form health survey: a general population application. In: Measuring Functioning and Well-Being: The Medical Outcomes Study Approach. Edited by AL Stewart, JE Ware. Durham, NC: Duke University Press, 1992; 277–90.

9. Ferrans C, Powers M. Quality of Life Index: development and psychometric properties. Adv Nurs Sci 1985; 8:15–24.

10. Warnecke R, Ferrans C, Johnson T, et al. Measuring quality of life in culturally diverse populations. J Nat Cancer Inst Monographs 1996; 20:29–38.

11. Eisen SV, Wilcox M, Leff HS, et al. Assessing behavioral health outcomes in outpatient programs: reliability and validity of the BASIS-32. J Behav Health Serv Res 1999; 26:5–17.

12. The EuroQoL Group. EuroQoL – a new facility for the measurement of health-related quality of life. Health Policy 1990; 16:199–208.

13. Brooks R. EuroQoL: the current state of play. Health Policy 1996; 37:53–72.

14. Hayhurst H, Palmer S, Abbott R, et al. Measuring health-related quality of life in bipolar disorder: relationship of the EuroQol (EQ-5D) to condition-specific measures. Qual Life Res 2006; 15:1271–80.

## Chapter 9: Assessment of pediatric bipolar disorder

1. Loranger AW, Levine PM. Age at onset of bipolar affective illness. Arch Gen Psychiatry 1978; 35:1345–8.

2. Joyce PR. Age of onset in bipolar affective disorder and misdiagnosis as schizophrenia. Psychol Med 1984; 14:145–9.

3. McGlashan TH. Adolescent versus adult onset of mania. Am J Psychiatry 1988; 145:221–3.

4. Geller B, Luby J. Child and adolescent bipolar disorder: a review of the past 10 years. J Am Acad Child Adolesc Psychiatry 1997; 36:1168–76.

5. Post RM, Leverich GS, Xing G, et al. Developmental vulnerabilities to the onset and course of bipolar disorder. Dev Psychopathol 2001; 13:581–98.

6. Achenbach TM. Integrative Guide for the 1991 CBCL/4–18, YSR, and TRF Profiles. Burlington, VT: University of Vermont, Department of Psychiatry, 1991.

7. Crijnen AAM, Achenbach TM, Verhulst FC. Problems reported by parents of children in multiple cultures: the Child Behavior Checklist syndrome constructs. Am J Psychiatry 1999; 156:569–74.

8. Nolan TM, Bond L, Adler R, et al. Child Behavior Checklist classification of behavior disorder. J Paediatr Child Health 1996; 32:405–11.

9. Fombonne E. The Child Behavior Checklist and the Rutter Parental Questionnaire: a comparison between two screening instruments. Psychol Med 1989; 19:777–85.

10. Youngstrom EA, Gracious BL, Danielson CK, et al. Toward an integration of parent and clinician report on the Young Mania Rating Scale. J Affect Disord 2003; 77:179–90.

11. Hudziak JJ, Althoff RR, Derks EM, et al. Prevalence and genetic architecture of Child Behavior Checklist-juvenile bipolar disorder. Biol Psychiatry 2005; 58:562–8.

12. Holtmann M, Bolte S, Goth K, et al. Prevalence of the Child Behavior Checklist-pediatric bipolar disorder phenotype in a German general population sample. Bipolar Disord 2007; 9:895–900.

13. Faraone SV, Althoff RR, Hudziak JJ, et al. The CBCL predicts DSM bipolar disorder in children: a receiver operating characteristic curve analysis. Bipolar Disord 2005; 7:518–24.

14. Volk HE, Todd RD. Does the Child Behavior Checklist juvenile bipolar disorder phenotype identify bipolar disorder? Biol Psychiatry 2007; 62:115–20.

15. Diler RS, Birmaher B, Axelson D, et al. The Child Behavior Checklist (CBCL) and the CBCL-bipolar phenotype are not useful in diagnosing pediatric bipolar disorder. J Child Adolesc Psychopharmacol 2009; 19:23–30.

16. Gracious BL, Youngstrom EA, Findling RL, et al. Discriminative validity of a parent version of the Young Mania Rating Scale. J Am Acad Child Adolesc Psychiatry 2002; 41:1350–9.

17. Shaffer D, Gould MS, Brasic J, et al. A children's global assessment scale (CGAS). Arch Gen Psychiatry 1983; 40:1228–31.

18. Endicott J, Spitzer RL, Fleiss JL, et al. The Global Assessment Scale: a procedure for measuring overall severity of psychiatric disturbance. Arch Gen Psychiatry 1976; 33:766–71.

19. Bird HR, Canino G, Rubio-Stipec M, et al. Further measures of the psychometric properties of the Children's Global Assessment Scale. Arch Gen Psychiatry 1987; 44:821–24.

20. Geller B, Warner K, Williams M, et al. Prepubertal and young adolescent bipolarity versus ADHD: assessment and validity using the WASH-U-KSADS, CBCL and TRF. J Affect Disord 1998; 51:93–100.

21. Geller B, Zimerman B, Williams M, et al. Reliability of the Washington University in St. Louis Kiddie Schedule for Affective Disorders and Schizophrenia (WASH-U-KSADS) mania and rapid cycling sections. J Am Acad Child Adolesc Psychiatry 2001; 40:450–5.

22. Geller B, Sun K, Zimerman B, et al. Complex and rapid-cycling in bipolar children and adolescents: a preliminary study. J Affect Disord 1995; 34:259–68.

23. Chambers WJ, Puig-Antich J, Hirsch M, et al. The assessment of affective disorders in children and adolescents by semi-structured interview: test-retest reliability of the Schedule for Affective Disorders and Schizophrenia for School-Age Children, Present Episode version. Arch Gen Psychiatry 1985; 42:696–702.

24. Geller B, Zimerman B, Williams M, et al. Six-month stability of a prepubertal and early adolescent bipolar disorder phenotype. J Child Adolesc Psychopharmacol 2000; 10:165–73.

## Chapter 10: Assessment of comorbidities

1. Kessler RC, McGonagle K, Zhao S, et al. Lifetime and 12 month prevalence of DSM-III-R psychiatric disorders in the United States. Results from the National Comorbidity Survey. Arch Gen Psychiatry 1994; 51:8–19.

2. Fajutrao L, Locklear J, Priaulx J, et al. A systematic review of the evidence of the burden of bipolar disorder in Europe. Clin Pract Epidemol Ment Health 2009; 5:3.

3. McElroy SL, Altshuler LL, Suppes T, et al. Axis I psychiatric comorbidity and its relationship to historical illness variables in 288 patients with bipolar disorder. Am J Psychiatry 2001; 158:420–6.

4. Vieta E, Colom F, Corbella B, et al. Clinical correlates of psychiatric comorbidity in bipolar I patients. Bipolar Disord 2001; 3:253–8.

5. Vieta E, Colom F, Martinez-Arán A, et al. Personality disorders in bipolar II patients. J Nerv Ment Dis 1999; 187:245–8.

6. Kaye W, Weltzin TE, Hsu LKG, et al. Patients with anorexia nervosa have elevated scores on Yale-Brown Obsessive Scale. Int J Eat Disord 1992; 12:57–62.

7. Simpson SG, al-Mufti R, Andersen AE, et al. Bipolar II affective disorder in eating disorder inpatients. J Nerv Ment Dis 1992; 180:719–22.

8. Vieta E, Colom F, Martínez-Arán A, et al. Bipolar II disorder and comorbidity. Compr Psychiatry 2000; 41:339–43.

9. Hudson JI, Pope HG, Jonas JM, et al. Phenomenologic relationship of eating disorders to major affective disorders. Psychiatric Res 1983; 9:435–54.

10. Goodwin FK, Jamison KR. Manic-Depressive Illness. New York: Oxford University Press, 1990.

11. Montejo J, Ayuso-Gutiérrez JL. Estacionalidad del trastorno bipolar. In: Trastornos Bipolares. Edited by E Vieta, C Gastó. Barcelona: Springer-Verlag, 1997; 291–311.
12. Wehr TA, Rosenthal NE. Seasonality and affective illness. Am J Psychiatry 1989; 146:829–39.
13. Kruger S, Shugar G, Cooke RG. Comorbidity of binge eating disorder and the partial binge eating syndrome with bipolar disorder. Int J Eat Disord 1996; 19:45–52.
14. Elmslie JL, Silverstone JT, Mann JI, et al. Prevalence of overweight and obesity in bipolar patients. J Clin Psychiatry 2000; 61:179–84.
15. Elmslie JL, Mann JI, Silverstone JT, et al. Determinants of overweight and obesity in patients with bipolar disorder. J Clin Psychiatry 2001; 62:486–91.
16. Fagiolini A, Frank E, Houck MSH, et al. Prevalence of obesity and weight change during the treatment in patients with bipolar I disorder. J Clin Psychiatry 2002; 63:528–33.
17. McElroy SL, Frye MA, Suppes T, et al. Correlates of overweight and obesity in 644 patients with bipolar disorder. J Clin Psychiatry 2002; 63:207–13.
18. Allison DB, Casey DE. Antipsychotic-induced weight gain: a review of the literature. J Clin Psychiatry 2001; 62:22–31.
19. Chengappa KN, Chalassani L, Brar JS, et al. Changes in body weight and body mass index among psychiatric patients receiving lithium, valproate, or topiramate: an open-label, non-randomized chart review. Clin Ther 2002; 24:1576–84.
20. Torrent C, Vieta E, Garcia-Garcia M. Validation of the Barcelona Bipolar Eating Disorder Scale for bipolar patients with eating disturbances. Psychopathology 2008; 41:379–87.
21. Fagiolini A, Kupfer DJ, Houck PR, et al. Obesity as a correlate of outcome in patients with bipolar I disorder. Am J Psychiatry 2003; 160:112–7.

## Chapter 11: Assessment of functioning

1. Rosa AR, Sanchez-Moreno J, Martinez-Aran A, et al. Validity and reliability of the Functioning Assessment Short Test (FAST) in bipolar disorder. Clin Pract Epidemol Ment Health 2007; 3:5.
2. Kauer-Sant'Anna M, Bond DJ, Lam RW, et al. Functional outcomes in first-episode patients with bipolar disorder: a prospective study from the Systematic Treatment Optimization Program for Early Mania project. Compr Psychiatry 2009; 50:1–8.
3. Fajutrao L, Locklear J, Priaulx J, et al. A systematic review of the evidence of the burden of bipolar disorder in Europe. Clin Pract Epidemol Ment Health 2009; 5:3.
4. Altshuler L, Tekell J, Biswas K, et al. Executive function and employment status among veterans with bipolar disorder. Psychiatr Serv 2007; 58:1441–7.
5. Weinstock LM, Miller IW. Functional impairment as a predictor of short-term symptom course in bipolar I disorder. Bipolar Disord 2008; 10:437–42.

## Chapter 12: Assessment of suicidality

1. Fajutrao L, Locklear J, Priaulx J, et al. A systematic review of the evidence of the burden of bipolar disorder in Europe. Clin Pract Epidemol Ment Health 2009; 5:3.
2. Osborn D, Levy G, Nazareth I, et al. Suicide and severe mental illnesses. Cohort study within the UK general practice research database. Schizophr Res 2008; 99:134–8.
3. Valtonen HM, Suominen K, Mantere O, et al. Suicidal behavior during different phases of bipolar disorder. J Affect Disord 2007; 97:101–7.

4.  Valtonen HM, Suominen K, Haukka J, et al. Differences in incidence of suicide attempts during phases of bipolar I and II disorders. Bipolar Disord 2008; 10:588–96.

5.  Simon GE, Hunkeler E, Fireman B, et al. Risk of suicide attempt and suicide death in patients treated for bipolar disorder. Bipolar Disord 2007; 9:526–30.

6.  Posner K, Oquendo MA, Gould M, et al. Columbia Classification Algorithm of Suicide Assessment (C-CASA): classification of suicidal events in the FDA's pediatric suicidal risk analysis of antidepressants. Am J Psychiatry 2007; 164:1035–43.

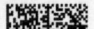